A Good Death

Conversations with East Londoners

Michael Young
and Lesley Cullen

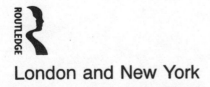

London and New York

First published 1996
by Routledge
11 New Fetter Lane, London EC4P 4EE

Simultaneously published in the USA and Canada
by Routledge
29 West 35th Street, New York, NY 10001

Routledge is an International Thomson Publishing company

© 1996 Institute of Community Studies

Phototypeset in Times
by Intype London Ltd
Printed and bound in Great Britain by Clays Ltd, St Ives PLC

British Library Cataloguing in Publication Data
A catalogue record for this book is available from the British Library

Library of Congress Cataloguing in Publication Data
Young, Michael Dunlop
   A good death : conversations with East Londoners / Michael Young
and Lesley Cullen
     p. cm.
   Includes bibliographical references and index.
   1. Terminal care—England—London. 2. Terminally ill—
England—London—Family relationships. 3. Terminally ill—
England—London—Psychology. 4. Cancer—Psychological aspects.
5. Death—Psychological aspects. 6. Bereavement—Psychological
aspects. 7. East End (London, England) I. Cullen, Lesley,
1945–   II. Title.
R726.8.Y675   1996
362.1′75′09421—dc20   95–25968
                                           CIP

ISBN 0–415–13796–9 (hbk)
ISBN 0–415–13797–7 (pbk)

A Good Death

Increasing numbers of people are now faced by the need, either
with terminal illnesses effectively cutting short time to contemplate
a ... death. ... Book is based on work of how
l ... people ... ways of incinating and helping
i ... death and surviving grief.
T ... conversations with people who are
t ... and with the doctors, nurses, and hos
p ... look after them

... book are mostly those of people who have
n ... despite being under the shadow of impending
d ... experience could be a comfort to others in a
s ... situation. A Good Death is intended for people who are
d ... the law and professional carers and for carers: doc
t ... nurses and social workers.

M ... Director at and **Lesley Ballor** is a Research
C ... and Community ... Young is
t ... with
P ...

For Sasha Moorsom

Contents

Preface
Personal note

At the time of going to press it is nearly two years since the death of my wife, Sasha. It is nearly two years, but to describe the actual event in that way does not seem at all right. It gets nearer to the feeling of it if I say 'since Sasha died'. It wasn't a death: Sasha died. After much delay I have been able to get back to the book. But my acceptance of what has happened is still spasmodic.

How much so was brought home to me again the other day by a vision in a London street. Crowds of people were shuffling along the pavements, past the shops, the pizzarias and McDonald's, and as I looked at them I didn't need to ask myself what their destination was. The thousands of us there would before long be dead – the whole lot of us – the old, the young, even the babies – not a single person would be left. Our descendants would be outside the shops perhaps, but none of us. For a moment the others seemed to be as much aware as I was of where we were marching to. Their faces became more grey, their heads dropped, their shoulders hunched. The colours in the shop windows faded. In the next moment they were no longer moving towards their destination. They had already reached it. They were already dead.

I wondered after the illusion had vanished why I had conjured it up and why it gripped me so tightly. Why was I so affected by the commonplace thought that the armies of shoppers, all the billions of people in the world for that matter, would soon be dead? It was not just the sadness of it; on the other side of the sadness was the sense of being at one – the atonement – with them. Also, as I had imagined that the people in the street were dead, and there was no distinction between the living and the dead, so Sasha might move back to the other side of the line and reappear. It is clear, if with decreasing credibility, that I am still trying, and will go on trying in what life is left to me, to deny that what has happened has happened. While knowing that the sightings of her, in the street or on the stairs at home, are halluci-nations, I also do not know; I am not sure.

Then I rediscovered the East Londoners whom Lesley Cullen and I had got to know before I had to abandon the book tempor-arily. With their valiant help I have been able, however hesitantly, to remember the sequence of events which led to Sasha's death. Most catastrophies are end-points but in a sequence; one way to make them less awful is to track back down the sequence, without too much varnishing by memory.

Sasha (she used her maiden name, Moorsom, for her novels, poems and sculptures) was as beautiful as when we'd met thirty-five years before. We were on holiday in France. The people around us in the streets there were not about to die.

Then her belly began to swell quickly and relentlessly. She could not be pregnant. She was 61. She was more uncomfortable each day. She could not eat. What was it? How much more could the skin stretch without bursting? In two days we hurried from holiday to incomprehension and gnawing fear. The French doctors we ran to had x-rays taken, prescribed tablets and looked con-cerned. The doctors in the local hospital would not tap off the liquid. They seemed (or pretended) to be as much in the dark as we were, and as many of the informants were in this book when they first realised that something serious was wrong.

On the Friday, I phoned the secretary of the surgeon at King's College Hospital in London who had recently operated on me for a secondary cancer in my liver. I had always comforted myself by thinking that I would die first. The secretary arranged for Sasha to be admitted on the Saturday if she could get back in time to see her GP beforehand. She flew back to England on the Friday night, and I broke all my records along the autoroutes from Marseilles Airport to King's almost in time to be there when she arrived on the Saturday afternoon.

She had been to her GP. Mercifully, and also dreadfully, the GP did not mince words. She said Sasha should not be surprised if it turned out she had ovarian cancer. We had both feared something of the sort without saying anything to each other. It was awful to know what the doctor thought. But the GP's open-ness allowed us to use the word, cancer. We felt as if we had been hit on the head with a hammer, and yet we were helped by being able to use the dreaded word about Sasha as we had learnt to use it about me.

When he saw her on the Monday my surgeon resignedly pronounced it was not his business, not her liver, and transferred her to Gynaecology. The liquid was produced by the tumour which had caused the abdomen to swell (a condition known as ascites). The liquid was drawn off, and then everything came to a stop. I had half expected (despite the experience of our informants) that, in what was an emergency for us, quick action would be taken before the cancer spread too far. There would be prompt surgery or other treatment. Not at all. Instead of that, Sasha was sent home to wait for the results of tests. To wait. To wait. To wait. We were in for many long periods of helpless waiting. Cancer is waiting. Slowly, agonisingly slowly, the results came in and a date was booked for the operation. We imagined the cancerous cells swimming ever deeper into her abdomen. We were already starting to become institutionalised, using doctors' words like abdomen.

Eventually, Sasha was operated on, and her uterus and various tumours removed. Surgery could not take out all the cancerous cells which were floating about. To follow up on the surgery and kill off as many of these cells as possible the best bet was a relatively new platinum-based drug, cisplatin. The sister in the ward said that we no longer need worry; cisplatin had revolutionised the prospects for women like Sasha. But as bad luck would have it, the operation left behind a wound which would not heal. There were a few weeks' delay before chemotherapy could begin. Other women from the ward who had been through the same operation at the same time as Sasha were able to start the chemotherapy very soon afterwards. We were jealous of them as they sat around at the end of the beds looking smug. We had to wait.

The surgeon said there was no point in Sasha starting on the further treatment at King's. Since we lived nearer to Barts it would be better to be transferred there. I could not follow the reasoning. It was life and death. What matter a few more minutes on the journey? A transfer would inevitably mean more waiting. We would again be caught up in delays. The papers from King's might not get through to Barts. They didn't. Nor did they get to the Homerton Hospital where Sasha was referred by Barts for her regular injections. Nor to the Royal Marsden Hospital for Cancer,

which was the last hospital Sasha went to a year later when all
else had failed.

There was an additional anxiety about Barts. The Tomlinson
Report had just been published. It proposed the closure of Barts.
We knew this would mean upheaval. There was nothing in Tomlinson about the extra pain for patients in a hospital which was
for the Bottomley chop. Why then was she to go from a hospital
which was not threatened to one that was? The surgeon shrugged
his shoulders. He was adamant. Sasha had to go. Perhaps he
thought the prognosis was too poor – the sort of suspicion that
patients cannot avoid – or just that our health authority would
have a contract with Barts but not with King's.

We were right about Tomlinson. It did put a blight on Barts.
Staff morale took a knock. Yet it gave me a chance to try and
do something and to distract myself (as I am always liable to do)
by busying myself over the closure. It took up some of the waiting
time to do as much as I could as President of the College of
Health to save Barts and Sasha together. On balance, Tomlinson
may have been good for my mental health though not for Sasha's.
Later on, when the Royal Marsden Hospital was threatened I
wrote to the Prime Minister and asked him how he would like it
if his wife had cancer and she could not be treated with some of
the drugs still on trial because the main specialist cancer hospital
in London had closed.

In my gullible state, what happened next I took to be a small
miracle assisted by poor staff work in Downing Street. I got a
letter back from Mr Major addressed in his own hand to 'Dear
David', with a postscript saying he hoped my wife was well and
that we would meet again before too long. I knew at once that I
had been mistaken for the other Lord Young, the real Lord
Young, Lord Young of Graffham, who had once been Secretary
of State for Trade and Industry in Mrs Thatcher's Cabinet. If the
Prime Minister's letter had been passed on to the Department of
Health it obviously would have carried a great deal more weight
than a hundred letters from me. As it happened, the Marsden
was reprieved, though I don't suppose either of the Lords Young
had anything to do with it, one wittingly, the other more influen-
tially but unwittingly.

Sasha never denied to herself that she had cancer, except in
her dreams. In her dreams she was never ill. But she used her
organising skills, not to tilt at Virginia Bottomley but to help a

distant relative, Anthony Scott. She felt he had received too little recognition as a composer of merit. From her bed she managed by means of countless letters to raise money – I think nearly £5,000 – for a concert of his music. From this she paid for first-class musicians and singers. She mobilised her family to distribute leaflets. The audience filled the great medieval church, the Church of St Bartholomew-the-Great, just by the hospital. Sasha came in a wheelchair, dressed in purple. Before and after the concert, she looked joyful at the centre of groups of friends.

The concert was only a month before she died and she may have known it was a kind of dress rehearsal for her funeral in the same church. At the funeral Ian Partridge sang again the song by Anthony Scott which he had dedicated to Sasha, with the words – *To His Sweet Saviour* – by Robert Herrick. A song – *Always in My Mind* – for which she herself had written words and music was also sung. She hoped that one day Cleo Laine might sing it.

Winter approaches
You are always in my mind
Maybe it's because the nights are colder now
Other winters, other times
We kept each other warm
A lonely night is a chill night
As winter approaches
And you
Are always in my mind.

When the spring comes
Will this winter ever end?
Every little thing brings back the memory
Of other winters, other times
When we were still together.
A cold night is a lonely night
No one to keep out the chill
As winter approaches
And you
Are always in my mind.

Before and after the concert was a terrible time for us, as the waiting was for the people in this book. We were being crushed between two sets of powers over which (despite my flutterings

over Tomlinson) we had no control – the seemingly implacable
disease within eating away the flesh in the recesses of her abdomen and the giant health service which, for all its marvels and
all its marvellous people, made us wait so long between one
appointment and another. But there were so many good times
too. It was worth having that final year after the holiday, particularly when my daughter, Sophie, came back home to stay. She
had been a Buddhist nun for eleven years.

It sometimes eased the pain to communicate between ourselves
in poetry. That autumn, not long after the race from Marseilles,
I wrote 'The Metronomic Moon'.

> In other years I would say, how pretty they are,
> The cherries outside our house.
> This autumn I see the first leaves
> Writhe from the green into the yellow and
> From the yellow into what seems frantic red
> Before they corkscrew to their conclusion
> When the morning wipers scrape them from the windscreens
> To drop them in the dog shit on the pavement
> Their beauty has not brought them mercy.
>
> The cherry flaunting first and shedding fastest
> Flies a few prayer flags in tatters.
> When the time is ripe (soon now)
> The metronomic moon on cue will let slip
> The north wind to bite the branches bare and
> Lay out the bony tree against the back-lit tombgrey sky.
> In other years I would say, how lucky we are,
> The people inside our house
> But the luck has not brought us mercy.

Sasha followed with 'Body'.

> What was so quiet a companion, my dumb friend,
> Now cries out, groans, swells up with noxious fluid
> Clamouring for attention.
> Did I neglect you? Taking for granted
> The ease with which you walked, breathed, ran for a bus?
> We that were one, are two.
> I bow before you.

And 'The Green Stone':

You are one and indivisible.
Mary, Kittisaro, stone,
I hold the green stone in my hand
And I am holding your two hands in mine.
Flesh dissolves, withers, burns
In the flame,
Ashes on the surface of the water like flower petals
Float downstream,
Our hands transformed to ashes;
Only the stone remains.

The poems about the cancer and other events in our lives were published as *Your Head in Mine*, Carcanet Press, 1994. Sophie wrote about 'The Green Stone' in her introduction to the book.

Sasha would sometimes use poetry to communicate in a more subtle way that which was difficult to talk about directly. This was the case with 'The Green Stone' which was written for two friends who had also recently left the monastic life, Mary and Kittisaro. On their last visit they had given her a green stone which she found very calming to hold in moments of pain or distress. This was just at the time when the second round of chemotherapy was stopped because it wasn't doing her any good. She knew then that she was dying. One evening after returning home from the hospital for the last time she showed me this poem. I read it sitting on her bed and realised that through these few lines of poetry she was telling me that she would soon be going and could accept with infinite sadness and yet peace this transformation of flesh to ashes. My eyes filled with tears and as we looked at each other there was an understanding deeper than any words could go.

I had taken the almost laughable course of setting up a National Funerals College to improve the conduct of funerals, and some of the ideas from that were introduced into Sasha's funeral. Sasha lay in an open coffin in the same church where she had sat in a wheelchair. The funeral director, Mr Cribb, invited each person to place a single flower on her body. There was music and poetry reading and chanting by brown-robed monks and talks by our two children, Toby as well as Sophie. The last poem of hers to be read was 'The Company of the Birds'.

Ah the company of the birds
I loved and cherished on Earth
Now, freed of flesh we fly
Together, a flock of beating wings,
I am as light, as feathery,
As gone from gravity we soar
In endless circles.

Afterwards in the cemetery there was a long silence amongst her
friends as Sasha's body was lowered into the grave. The human
silence was filled with the singing of what seemed like a chorus
of innumerable birds.

In the next long afterwards, up to now, there have been other
illusions and hallucinations besides the armies of the dead in the
street. The dead are dead and not dead. Sasha may have died,
but she is certainly not dead, and with this testament I declare
to the readers what will already be obvious – that I am very far
from being a dispassionate student of dying and of death.

Michael Young

Chapter 1

Slow death

The greatest triumph of the century is to have added twenty-five years to the average expectation of life or, to put it another way, subtracted twenty-five years from the expectation of death. There are more people still alive in their seventies and eighties – the number of people in the UK at 80 and over nearly trebled between 1951 and 1988, from 0.7 to 2.0 million, and even centenarians have multiplied.[1] This caps all that was done previously to extend life. But there has also been an increase in the numbers of people with a disabling or chronic disease[2] or a terminal, though lingering illness, whose lives have been prolonged by medical science. The dramatic postponement of death for the generality means more people who, because of their frailty, can hardly avoid thinking about the prospect of their own death. More people are around who can give an account of how they, and their carers, face death.

Hence this study. We hoped to get from patients themselves, and not from the doctors who are the experts, first-hand accounts of how they fared in the period leading up to their deaths, and from their survivors accounts of what happened to them afterwards. What did patients and their carers do when they could no longer cling to the presumption of continuing life which is the everyday comfort of the secular world? To get some ideas about the answers, we chose cancer patients for our enquiry. They were, and are, of special interest because their numbers are increasing, and are expected to continue doing so. 'The ageing of the population alone means that the overall number of new cancer patients will increase at an estimated 0.5% a year over the next 20 years.'[3]

For people who hope to have a quick death[4] – here today, gone tomorrow – the incidence of drawn-out deaths is little short of a disaster. But there is now a view about that a slow death is a better death than a quick one. This is not being advanced on the traditional grounds that the immortal soul could be in danger if people died so suddenly that they had no time to be shriven and make their peace with God. You could not die well unless you were spared long enough to do that and medieval treatises on how to do it once went into elaborate detail.[5] Not many people would now want to think that the road to heaven was paved with so many pitfalls that only with such precise instructions could one hope to avoid them. But a contemporary case for the slow death can still be made out on other grounds, as a modern cancer specialist has done. On one occasion, when he was asked to choose his preferred cause of death, he opted unhesitatingly for cancer. He was with a group of other people at the time.

> Most of them in fact chose to die very suddenly of a heart attack. I think a large part of it may be due to misconceptions people have about cancer, the feeling that people have that it's a prolonged and painful and awful death, something that anybody looking after a cancer patient knows simply isn't true for the great majority of patients. Many people don't have pain and those that do can almost always have it well controlled with modern medication. From my point of view I don't see it in such a negative context, perhaps because I am used to dealing with cancer patients and don't suffer from all the misconceptions that other people have. But I can actually see a lot of advantages, an advantage to having a chance to be able to come to terms with dying and with yourself, other people, to sort things out in your life over a period of time; to round off your life.[6]

He could also have referred to the grief of the survivors. Several studies have suggested that for them a sudden death is far more difficult to get over than a death which can be anticipated and prepared for.[7]

Whatever the pros and cons of a slow death, there is no reason to think it is not here to stay. It will become less and less possible to hold the idea, even in the back of your mind, that you are in some way exempt from death if growing numbers of people are most obviously not; and if they are around to say so in no uncertain terms. What then? Will that just add to fear? Or will people in such numbers, who cannot any longer cling to the attitudes typical of the hale and the hearty, move away from the denial of death and towards an acceptance of it in a new way? If they do, will it also move the whole culture so as to make it more friendly to death?

To throw some light on such questions cancer patients were suitable for three main reasons. The first is that, as we have been saying, most cancer deaths are slow. Although cancer is still terrifying, it is not quite so much so, due partly to the surgery which removes some cancers and to the general improvements in treatment which have increased the time between diagnosis and death. As a result, increasing numbers of people (like our informants) have the disease and yet have not been laid completely low by it. Their names are not struck off electoral registers or records in social benefit agencies. They get about and they have time to talk. They remain members of society but, knowing they have an ordinarily fatal disease, unless they deny it completely and put it out of their minds, they cannot altogether avoid reflecting a good deal on what is going to happen.

The first reason – the slowing down of cancer deaths – would not have been enough without the second reason, that cancer can now be talked about relatively openly. Not so long ago it could only be mentioned in hushed tones, and then often only by using one of a range of euphemisms – tumour, swelling, inflammation. It was the Big C,[8] a mystery without known cause or cure, an omen of death like the sign painted on the doors of the victims of the Great Plague who were nailed into their houses so that they had to stay there until they died. Cancer was the modern plague, even thought by many to be infectious. It is sometimes still thought to be so. One of our informants said she felt like a leper when a friend would not drink from a coffee cup she had used earlier lest she 'catch' cancer. Nevertheless, there has been a big change.

The third reason for our choice is that cancer patients, or anyone else with a fatal but lingering illness, need to be cared for, and, if they have families, will usually be looked after by them. There was thus a link with previous work at the Institute of Community Studies, where the present study was made, and particularly with two about widowhood. Peter Marris showed, in what came to be regarded as a classic study of the subject, that the general health of widows was worse than before bereavement.[9]

A few years later it was postulated that members of families keep each other alive, the form of the proposition being that one death within a family hastens another. A sample of just under 4,500 widowers was chosen to test the hypothesis – in this way the opposite of this present intensive study of a few people which can at best do no more than suggest hypotheses. Amongst the 4,500, it was shown that the death rate increased by 40 per cent in the first six months of bereavement before gradually dropping back to the mortality rate for married men of the same age.[10] This led to further work by other researchers in the USA, Sweden and elsewhere which found the same broad result.

A follow-up study of the same 4,500 people made by Parkes and colleagues showed that three-quarters of the increased death rate was attributable to heart disease.[11] It is spot-on when people talk about dying of a 'broken heart', as they did long before any systematic research was done. In a further follow-up in the unlikely place of Papua, New Guinea, amongst the Huli people, the increased death rate was shown to be greater amongst widowers than widows, and all studies made elsewhere have shown the same sex difference. The suggestion for New Guinea was that this difference might be due to the therapeutic effect of women (but not men) being encouraged to mourn in the 'crying house' and to denounce the dead person for dying.[12] This present study also follows two Institute reports on aspects of 'time', the first being about the way time is managed or mismanaged in a technological society, and the second about older people in the Third Age who have not yet had a terminal date put upon them.[13]

Method of study

The enquiry was shaped by the extent of our resources. It did not prove easy to attract funds. We did not have enough to allow us to draw a large and more representative sample. But we were able to obtain small, though indispensable and most welcome, grants from the Gulbenkian and Nuffield Foundations and from the Hilden Trust and these allowed us to set about, and maintain, the study.

Twelve people were referred to us by the major hospice in East London, St Joseph's.[14] It is close to the office of the Institute.

St Joseph's is one of the oldest hospices (set up in 1905) in a series of remarkable institutions which have grown in number mostly in the second half of the century. After our research design had been cleared by the hospital's Ethics Committee, two people came from the equally near Royal London Hospital. What we asked was that we should be put in touch with people who, in the view of the doctors and nurses, had (1) between three and four months to live, (2) could be seen at home, and (3) would be willing to talk to us. We will touch in turn on each of these requirements and their consequences for our research. To preserve confidentiality, the names of informants have been altered and a few other details changed.

Terminally ill

The reckoning turned out to be rather accurate, at any rate for the majority. Only three of the people lived longer than six months after we were first introduced to them, but these three confounded the doctors by a good margin and altered our time-table for the study – Julia Searle lived for eleven months, Harold Allen for a year and Kenneth Chandler for three years. We saw each of them as frequently as they would allow, and went on until they died, and then continued to see the relatives for a further year or more. The number who could be seen in any month, and the number of new patients who could be taken on but only when previous ones had died, was limited by the time that the two of us (being part time on the project) could put in during the interviewing period from October 1988 to the end of 1992, except for Kenneth and his widow who were seen for nearly two years after that. Lesley Cullen did most of the interviewing. We did not decide at the beginning to include only fourteen people in the study. We continued to take on new people (but only as others dimed) whom we could manage within a period of four years or so, and the number turned out to be fourteen. The work was delayed because the cancer which Michael Young had had recurred in another part of his body and his wife also developed cancer and died of it while the study was in progress.

The number of interviews with an individual and his or her survivors varied considerably. The people who lived longer, and whose bereaved relatives and friends were ready to be visited, were naturally seen more than others. At one extreme Alice

Colyer was seen three times and Arthur Jacobs four times; at the other, Julia Searle and her friend were interviewed on thirty-eight occasions, Kenneth and Florence Chandler on thirty-three and Harold and Lilian Allen on twenty-five. There is, of course, more to say about the people who were seen more often.

All the people were in the terminal stages of their illness as the doctors calculated (or miscalculated) it. But the accounts we were given were of the whole illness since its beginning. Some people had been ill for longer – this being in part due to the kind of cancer they had.[15]

The three women with breast cancer lived for thirteen, eleven and four years respectively after it had been diagnosed, whereas the three people with lung cancer all died within a year of diagnosis. Those with breast cancer were rivalled for longevity as a group only by two of the men, Dermot Donoghue, who had had a skin cancer on his face since 1986, and Kenneth Chandler, whose cancer of the bladder was first diagnosed in 1986 and who did not die until the autumn of 1992. His cancer was not his only problem by any means. The others, with other cancers, did not live so long. The shortest time for anyone between diagnosis and death was nine months. Judged by the standards of the past, before medical technology had advanced to its present state, people in the enquiry had slow deaths.

The patients had not been told that their doctors thought they had between three and four months to live. It would have been greatly resented by most of them if they had, and would have been wrong anyway. They were told we were making a study of people with serious illnesses like theirs and how they managed at home. It was part of our understanding with St Joseph's that we should not say anything about the prognosis. We could not, therefore, ask direct questions about death. People told us a great deal about their attitude to it but not in response to our questions. There were many questions we would have liked to ask, but could not. We were listeners and observers, not interrogators.

Seen at home

The patients were all at home and mostly being visited by members of the St Joseph's Home Care Team, which will be referred to in the text as Home Care Team or Home Care nurses.[16] The East End is one of the parts of the country where a home care service (as it is also sometimes called) operates rather intensively. It consists of specially trained nurses, doctors and social workers who give to some terminally ill patients at home broadly the same kind of support and the same means of controlling pain that they would get if they were in the hospice. So our people were receiving good physical care at home; this was helpful for the study as it threw into higher relief some of the issues around people's states of mind.

We wanted to see people at home rather than in a hospital or hospice. We thought it would be more conducive to the sort of conversations we hoped to have, and we would have a better chance of getting to know the carers. The hospice Home Care Team (called Macmillan nurses by some of our informants) gave us the opportunity we needed.

Willing to talk

The last criterion by which we chose our subjects, or they chose us, is almost too obvious to be worth mentioning. We do so because, more than anything else, it may have determined who our collaborators were. The people, including the carers, had to be willing, even want, to talk to us, which not everyone was who was approached on our behalf by a nurse or social worker. The staff at St Joseph's said that the people they selected for us were not all that unusual.

We are naturally enough very much in the debt of our informants. They were generous with their time, of which they did not have much left, and so were the carers. The staff of the hospice were invariably helpful. Dr Hanratty, Medical Director when the study began, Dr Heyse-Moore, Medical Director later, Dr G. Zeppetella, Consultant in Palliative Medicine and Dorothy Poing-destre, Senior Social Worker, were most helpful. Sheila Thompson was the senior social worker at the hospice when we began, and when she retired she became a valuable adviser to us. Dr Colin Murray Parkes, who has written so well about our subject, first set us on the road and gave us valuable criticisms. Prudence Smith worked over and criticised the draft in her wonderfully meticulous way.

We would also like to thank: Nicholas Albery, Paul Barker, Ann and Don Benton, Ann Cartwright, Stanley Cribb, Geoff Dench, Sister Denholm, Mary Douglas, Father Evan-Jones, Father

John Farrell, Charles Fletcher, Tony Flower, Kate Gavron, A.H. Halsey, Father Michael Hollings, Mr E.R. Howard, Canon Paul Jobson, Malcolm Johnson, Rev. Peter Jupp, Peter Laslett, Dr Rosemary Lennard, Dayan Lichtenstein, Shirley Lunn, Ian McColl, Monica Malone, Julia Neuberger, Father O'Connor, Chris Phillipson, Dr David Rampton, Marianne Rigge, Dave Robins, Rev. Fred Rollinson, Hilary Rubinstein, St Christopher's Hospice Information Service, Clive Seale, Rev. Bob Stephen, Nigel Wallace-Smith, Tony Walter, Roger Warren-Evans, Dr J.M. Waterhouse, Peter Willmott, Phyllis Willmott, Sophie Young and, above all, Wyn Tucker for keeping the office going and Sue Chisholm for typing and reproducing a shaming number of drafts.

Many others whom we saw and many authors whose books and papers we read gave us guidance. It has been said that when you copy one other writer that is plagiarism; when you copy many others, that is research. In that sense our work is research.

We hardly need say that fourteen people in East London, and their survivors, who may be untypical, are far too few to permit any generalisations. We did not see them for that purpose. We chose them (or rather they were chosen for us) as individuals who might be able to throw some light on large issues and in discussing these issues we have presented the same individuals in different contexts even though it involves a certain amount of repetition. We have also taken account of other studies, other information and other ideas as well. The patients certainly cannot be dismissed because they are not experts. Any person whosoever can have as much understanding of death as any other. An ex-docker in Wapping can have as much insight as an ex-archbishop, or even a present one. We are all fumbling. For all of us who cannot know anything for sure, death is the ground on which the whole world can speculate in common. It is also the ground on which we can stand together, to support each other, and show to each other, especially to the dying and the bereaved, that our minds and spirits are with them, that neither they nor (we hope) we die alone.

Chapter 2

The patients

We now introduce the individual people. For none of them was their life without incident. For long stretches, while they were in bed, or sitting in a chair, time could move slowly enough. But if they were, as never before, on the alert to interrogate the bodies which had brought them such an unwelcome new interest, at least it was an interest and one which gave the utmost scope for sometimes painful learning. Their bodies were no longer the silent, uncomplaining companions they had once been. Their bodies had turned traitor. Their bodies were making themselves felt, or it was feared they would before long; or if they were already in a bad patch they could look forward to, or at any rate hope for, some relief to come.

Apart from their common interest, the most obvious similarity between the fourteen people was that they were less their own masters and mistresses than they had been. At the time when we saw them they no longer had jobs which they had to go out to every day. They no longer had the round of little daily duties which in ordinary times hardly seem duties at all. Much as they would have liked to, they did not have to do shopping or as much of the work around the house as before. But in place of these, the everyday while-aways which make the healthy so busy, they were surrounded by a whole new set of constraints, generally much tighter than those they had displaced. From the time that the illness took hold, and increasingly as it bit deeper, their lives were more under the dominion of inescapables, of external forces that were beyond their own control, with death itself looming over all.

Some of these forces did not bear heavily on them at all, nor helped them, being to do with what was happening in society at large and were hardly any more under the control of their own doctors than of themselves. There were the advances in medicine brought about as the result of a world-wide cooperation between scientists, technologists and doctors. There was the growth of hospices as new institutions specifically designed to look after people recognised to be dying. There was the beginning of a new attitude (as we shall see in the next chapter) on the part of doctors. All this, and more, was, while happening well beyond East London, affecting it deeply, and changing the nature of dying there as elsewhere.

The people were less their own masters and mistresses because they were caught up in a common process from which in the longer run there was no escape. Once within what is aptly called the system, of high-tech and highly specialised medicine, they went through all the standard procedures of being examined, tested, diagnosed, treated and re-treated and, since it was all done within the National Health Service, without being charged for it. With a readiness which shows people's astonishing adapt-ability and credulity, they fell into the new role of patient as if they'd known all along what they should do when in fact they were imitating other patients around them who were all in turn doing what the doctors expected of them, or what they imagined the doctors expected of them. The powerful docker and the indomitable mother became equally meek, almost as if they were hiding their existence when they put their heads round the door of the consulting room or when the consultant swept around the ward with his retinue. Seldom assertive, the patients were mostly the passively obedient creatures of the system and all its marvel-lous works, which to a large extent dominated their lives from that time on. By submitting to what was done to them, while also vigorously asserting their independence, they were to all intents and purposes attempting to prolong their lives even while there was a contraction in what they could do with them. Not all were as pliant. But for most people the new pattern of their lives was largely determined from outside. The series of medical inter-ventions to which they were subject introduced a special kind of wave motion into their existence.

The ups followed a successful treatment and the downs came when the effect of it wore off. There was no straight-line decline from high points of health to the low-point of death; more usually there were several returns to relative health when the growth of the cancer was, temporarily, arrested or for a time reversed. Several people started off with major surgery which was followed, at different intervals and sometimes repeatedly, by chemotherapy and radiotherapy. The decline was punctuated and checked by the successive treatments, and the intervals between the treatments tended to get shorter as time went on. The rhythms operated rather as breathing goes in and out but with a breath lasting for months or years instead of seconds. The rise and fall was partially predictable. The doctors knew what the effect of their treatment was likely to be and roughly how long the relief would last. But, again, they only knew that for the average patient and, fortunately, not for any of the particular patients whom they or we saw.

Much of this treatment had been given before we came on the scene. Some people recounted the history of their illness when it was almost over. But they never tired of telling us their whole story once again, starting from a fateful Friday, or Monday or Tuesday – they could nearly always remember the day of the week, and sometimes even the hour, when they had their first serious symptoms or the first frightening encounter with a doctor.

All the patients were caught up in a temporal relationship with doctors and the best way of showing how much this matters is to give a couple of examples. Dermot is the first.[1]

Dermot Donoghue (51)[2]

Colon cancer. Single, living in Bow. An Irish loner with a charming young man's smile and a lightness to him. He was separated early in his life from his parents. A man of few words, he always pauses before answering a question. Until taken ill, he worked as a kitchen porter in London. He is always thirsty.

Dermot Donoghue had his first hospital visit on a day in October 1986.

October 1986   GP referred Dermot to London Hospital
                      where a biopsy was done. He had a cancer
                      on his face. Two weeks later radiotherapy was

begun. He attended every day for a ten-minute session for six months which involved having plastic eyeshades inserted into his eyes for protection. He had much pain and suffered sickness and diarrhoea. He gave up work because with the pain in his body he couldn't manage heavy lifting. He had to wear a bandage over his face and head which made him embarrassed to go out of doors.

October 1987

He suffered severe stomach pains and passed brown water. Ellen, a neighbour, called an ambulance and he was taken to the casualty department at the same hospital; he was admitted for tests. He was in hospital four to five weeks, and in the third week had an operation. Following that he felt much worse – he didn't feel at all prepared for what it would be like. Told he had a tumour behind the bowel which might return in six months to a year.

September 1988

A repeat of what happened the previous year with a second admission, more tests and another operation in the second week of his stay. He was 'starved' in the first week with a drip and water. He was told: 'this is the last time we can cut you up.' 'They're very quick to get you out ... I could have done with another two weeks both times.' During this stay a lady from the Macmillan Unit in the hospital visited him and had a chat and then referred him to St Josephs. Home Care nurses started visiting him at home after his discharge.

November 1988

We were introduced. Dermot was suffering from rectal carcinoma and widespread secondaries; he was very thin, emaciated, a picture of sadness and suffering. It was expected that he would eventually go into the hospice but for the present he was staying at home because he wanted to be near his neighbour and to have Christmas dinner with her as he had done for many years. She would be on her own except for a completely bedridden lady next door. Dermot had no other people in his life.

December 1988   Attacks of severe pain. He was admitted once again to the London where it was recommended he had a colostomy. He was in anguish about the prospects of another operation because of what had happened before. Had difficulty making the decision. There was no help or advice for him to draw on. He saw no other colostomy patients.

December 1988   Operation on 20 December. Woke up still in pain and in a ward isolated from the rest of the hospital because of an infection. If it continued, he would not be able to go into the hospice. Dermot spoke of a sudden awareness of what death meant; speaking about it before wasn't real.

January 1989   Still on Benson Ward all alone.

January 1989   Hospice suddenly made aware that Dermot had packed his bags and felt obliged to find him a bed quickly. Hospice became a family to one who never really knew family life.

February 1989   Dermot died at the hospice and was taken back to Ireland for burial with his family.

Dora Anstey (74)

Lung cancer. Widow in Haggerston with three daughters, Jackie, Debbie and Muriel. We first meet her in high summer when the weather is hot and white roses in a vase by her side are drooping. She does not notice the heat; she is cold enough to wear a mohair waistcoat and still keeps rubbing her arms to bring some warmth into them.

Dora's engagement with the system did not last so long as Dermot's.

October 1988	Had a cold and a long-lasting cough and went to GP but cough did not improve.
December 1988	Very poorly one day. GP visited and arranged admission to hospital. Kept there until mid-February the next year. A tumour was found a week after admission; an operation never considered. In January Dora had chemo-therapy, lost a lot of weight, was very ill and nearly died.
February 1989	Discharged back home. Home Care nurses came once a week and the doctor visited as well as social workers. Hospital check-ups once a month. Got better around Easter.
June 1989	We are introduced. Home Care nurses coming once every two weeks and continue to do so. Doctors at hospital noticed a slight deterio-ration shown by the x-ray at last visit. Very frail, doesn't go out alone because of fear of falling.
July 1989	Hospital visit in late June. Advised to have five radiotherapy treatments which have to be given in University College Hospital. 'I just can't believe it's happening. You think it's going to happen to other people, not yourself.'
August 1989	Frail and breathless. Planning to go away with friends for two weeks to Spain and looking forward to it. Hospital says she doesn't need more radiotherapy and can go if she wants. GP still calling once every one or two weeks and Hospice Home Care nurse once every two weeks.
August 1989	Daughters called Dora's GP because worried. GP advises not to go on holiday and Dora retires to her bedroom. She lost weight and got worse but was not in physical pain.
September 1989	Dora admitted to hospice where she died.

The Kübler-Ross stages

Once they were caught up in institutionalised medicine, the patients went backwards and forwards between hospital and home. Along with the fairly definite (though interrupted) growth and spread of cancer in the body, is there any parallel trajectory, not necessarily connected with medical treatments, in the inner life of people? The question has been studied before, most famously by Dr Kübler-Ross, one of the pioneers of the 'dignity in death' movement in the United States. Her influence, and that of the US experience, have affected practice in Britain just as British hospices have affected practice in the United States. The care of cancer patients has been almost as much a matter of international cooperation as the advances in treatment.

Dr Kübler-Ross has suggested five identifiable stages through which patients must pass before they can reach a final stage of acccptance.[3] They are *denial and isolation*, an essential protective stage dealing with the initial shock: it is characterised by 'selective hearing' by patients so they don't have to deal with too much too quickly. Our comment on this is that the initial denial can be extended into continued, intermittent denial of the sort experienced by many of our patients and by one of the authors of this book. It is followed by *anger*, often against those nearest to the patient, such as doctors or relatives, and sometimes against the patient's own self too. Kübler-Ross suggests the absence of anger indicates a possible lack of acceptance of the diagnosis. This is followed by *bargaining*, when patients attempt to extend their life expectancy by making deals (for example, with God or fate). *Depression* is the fourth stage and arises from the cumulative losses, physical and social, experienced by patients. Then 'if a patient has had enough time ... and has been given some help in working through the previously described stages, he will reach a stage during which he is neither depressd nor angry about his "fate"' (p. 99). This *acceptance* is not a happy stage but one 'almost void of feelings'. The stages were presented as succeeding each other in time with a certain sequential unfolding to them.

We met patients late in their illness and could only take a view from their recollections of what had happened before; their recollections are bound to have been edited by them, as recollections always are. But we have to say, to judge by what they told us, that these patients had not by and large followed the Kübler-

Ross sequences and, in particular, what we learned from them called into question any such scheme which does not give due weight to age. 'Our' patients more closely fitted what Murray Parkes has said:

> Others might (and probably will) adopt a different terminology when describing the phases through which the dying patient passes in the course of his illness. Since individual variation is so great, it is unlikely that any one conceptual system could be applied to all.[4]

What stood out from our patients was just that individual variation. The difference between the Kübler-Ross patients and ours may have been due in part to ours being at home. Since the former were seen in a hospital, what she may have been observing was not dying in general but the effects of institutionalisation. Walter has pointed this out.[5] Denial, anger, bargaining, depression, acceptance are precisely the way different people respond to incarceration in a total institution, leading to what Goffman terms mortification of the self.[6]

One patient – Jennifer – did seem to go through four of the five stages, and in succession, but in this respect she was unique amongst the fourteen.

Jennifer Barnes (56)

Afro-Caribbean nurse in Newham. Married. One son, Lee. Cancer of the pancreas. She looks tired as well as elegant as she moves her long limbs slowly and carefully. Her husband, John, has given up his work so that he can look after her.

Jennifer spent the first 24–36 hours after having been told her diagnosis in a state of shock which was no less because, as a nurse, she had had experience of giving the same news to other patients. It might be described as denial because she was unable to handle the information she was given and could not remember the substance of conversations with her doctors.

> On the Wednesday I didn't take it in and on the Thursday, it was worse. I went completely blank.

This was followed by a time of intensive talking with family and friends which seemed to help Jennifer without helping her family. When we met, she was still angry at the loss of her future. Until her death she remained a firm Christian, taking communion every week, but she did not seem to strike any 'bargains' with God. She was depressed and treated for it. In a short while the depression lifted as Jennifer found more satisfying roles for herself at home and started going out to see people rather than waiting for them to come to her.

Kübler-Ross distinguishes between reactive depression arising from past losses and preparatory depression when the person looks to impending losses and leaving this life. Several patients talked to us of the cumulative losses of job, companionship and their own familiar body, and expressed regrets, but not to the point of depression. Some of the changes they spoke of had happened so long ago or been handled in such a way that it seemed they had been successfully accommodated. A few patients were notably resilient in the face of repeated setbacks. Kenneth Chandler was one of them.

Kenneth Chandler (67)

Cancer of the bladder. Isle of Dogs. Married to Florence with four loving daughters, Linda, Karen, Sandra and Christine. Enough ailments to kill a regiment yet still with the carriage of a light-weight boxer. A war hero, he leaps to his feet whenever we come into the room and stands erect for a minute, as though he has a metal plate for a back instead of a backbone, almost in parody of the soldier he once was.

He had endured with robust spirit a series of setbacks, numbering among them an amputation of a leg after being shot on the Normandy beaches and three open heart operations. He almost seemed to thrive on it. He had not let misfortune get him down before, and he was not going to let the cancer do it, not while there was still even a remote chance that, with his determination, he might win a reprieve.

As for bargaining, if one gives a broad meaning to it, then

many of our people engaged in it and often. Carol seemed to be one who did.

Carol Taylor (39)

Breast cancer. Lives in Plaistow with her 18-year-old daughter, Diane, and her mother, Mary Champion, who has moved in to look after her. Carol is an attractive divorcee, slim and neatly dressed in a bright orange track-suit and matching turban to mask the loss of her fine blonde hair. Carol had lost her brother and her elder sister to cancer.

Carol made her body over to the teaching hospital where she was a patient to do with as they wished; she may have been hoping that in return for the gift of herself she would get some gifts back. But most instances of bargaining were much more explicit than that. It was quite common to make a pact that, if a person could live until a hoped for event actually happened, they would after that be ready to accept, even submit to, whatever fate had in store for them. There is more about that in Chapter 3.

Amongst the patients, acceptance was not dependent on moving through any set stages. Sheer exhaustion required people to withdraw from interaction with family and friends away from home and then, later, at home as well. Harold Allen did this.

Harold Allen (75)

Cancer of the pancreas. Married to Lilian, with two sons, Michael and Richard, and a daughter, Barbara. Has a wonderfully caring GP, Dr Clayton, who is important in Harold's story. A tall gaunt man who sometimes still looks like the soldier he once was. Lilian and he are both glad they stayed in Forest Gate, in the same district where they were brought up as children. The house suits them too, and the garden with its dense population of home-made gnomes.

Harold said, nearing the end, nine months after we began seeing him, 'Everything's going now. I can't think. I've not got any memory any more. I sit here all day and it's just nothing, you know.'

Kenneth Chandler was another patient similar in this respect. Three months before he died he noticed how he was 'turning in on himself', as others could notice from the look in his eyes he could feel himself withdrawing from people and said, 'I don't want to be like that. I want to be like my old self but it takes me over.'

Their families

Another respect in which most of the patients were the same was that they had families. While many of their friends had dropped away, it was family that tended to remain and so the book is to quite a large extent a family study. Perhaps almost everyone who has ever been married and had children hopes, if they think about it at all, that if they die first they will in their last days be looked after by their husband or wife, aided by their children. Men who know how much shorter their lives customarily are than those of their wives can assume that they will die first and look forward to this domestic ideal with a bit more confidence, unless they have wrecked their chances by parting decisively from the women who might, if they had been able to persevere, have become their nurses. There may be some slight compensation for their shorter lives if someone is there at home to see them off, or at least to visit them regularly in hospital or hospice until the end.[7]

If they had known what happens to cancer patients, they might have worked even more strenuously for this outcome. For a quick death it would not matter so much being alone. But if it has to be slow, let it at least be shared. Being alone with cancer is like a bad dream which the dreamer hopes will never happen in real life. But it happens, and on a very large scale, especially to older women, most especially to older women who were the youngest children and whose siblings are therefore likely to be dead. It is liable to happen whenever dying is long and drawn out. If all deaths were quick, they could mostly be in hospitals and hospices. The costs could be bearable. But not slow deaths. If all cancer and other dying patients had to be in hospital throughout their illness, there would be no room for anyone else, the Exchequer would be bankrupt and the National Health Service the National Dying Service. But it is not like that. In the intervals between visits to hospital the patient has to be somewhere and there is nowhere except home, which is where people want to be anyway, where human decencies can be preserved as much as possible. There is no choice except for a person expected to die within days or even hours, when it is not thought suitable for a person without anyone with them to die at home, although of course that happens too.

Whether or not our informants had anyone with them was even more beyond their control than what happened in the hospital, and could matter as much to their wellbeing. We go into more detail about this in Chapter 4, but it should be said now that the presence of a family, boon though it was to many, was not an unadulterated one. It depended on the situation of the family. Relations with relations could get more tense through a period when everyone was tired and having to adapt to profound changes in their everyday lives and in the stirring of their deepest feelings.

So much, as always, depends on expectations. At a low level, anticipating nothing, people could seem surprisingly accepting, whereas others with a relatively rich family life could be disappointed if it did not live up to their more demanding expectations. But for most people membership of a family was an asset. The studies referred to in the previous chapter showed that one death, of one family member, can bring on another. The other way round, there is some evidence that the presence of a family and good relations within it can keep people alive. According to one study of cancer patients:

> Patients who lived significantly longer tended to maintain co-operative and mutually responsive relationships, especially towards the end of their lives.[8]

Even when there is tension within a family, that may be conducive to survival. People keep each other alive by giving them something to live for.[9] This is obvious in every hospital ward. Visitors are what patients wait for, and cherish, and the sad ones are those who have none. One of the advantages of the more flexible visiting hours introduced in the last twenty years is that it is less painfully obvious who has no visitors. 'They' may always be coming later.

Age

People were mostly alike in having families but not in their ages, another factor which shapes the kind of deaths they had. It would be surprising if this were not so, if only because age is one of the cardinal principles by which behaviour is governed in our society.[10] Age is the cage we are forced into from the time when as children we are required by law to go to school at 5 until 16. In an age-stratified society people are under pressure to take a long view, at any rate of their working lives. A career, however much it straddles different occupations, has always to be marked out in relation to age until it suddenly ends at 60 or 65. It would be odd indeed, when so much is made of it, if thoughts of death were not mixed up with thoughts of age. Whatever their age, and however assiduously they try to blank out thoughts of death, no-one can forget that as they get older they are more likely to die, and that if they last out into a ripe old age they are eventually certain to. As Edgar says in *King Lear*:

> Men must endure
> Their going hence, even as their coming hither:
> Ripeness is all.[11]

Nor, as they get older, can they fail to ask themselves, perhaps rather frequently, how much longer they have.

Calculations can be elaborate according to people's state of health at particular periods in their lives; the ages at which their parents, and perhaps grandparents, died; the biblical three score years and ten; the ages at which friends have died; their knowledge of general expectations of life, all leading to a view of what is a ripe old age. Whatever the calculations, old age has one sealed-in tendency: to recede. It is nearly always older than you are. To a teenager 40 may seem old indeed, but not to a person who reaches that age, or likewise 60 or 70. Old age is the age you have not yet reached, a little older than you are, at least until such pretensions are so absurd they can no longer be preserved and it has to be accepted that you are lucky to have lived so long and that you can no longer complain with any show of reason that your life has been cut short.

It is therefore not surprising that there was a difference between the older and younger in our enquiry. The cancers the older people suffered from were no less deadly than those besetting the younger, but the older were in some ways not laid quite so low by the disease.[12] If you know yourself to be at an age by which many people would be dead, and so are almost at the point where you can realistically expect to be joining them before long, you cannot possibly believe you are not going to die at all, or, more modestly, that you still have a very long lease of life ahead. If you do not die of cancer you are going, before long, to die of something else, and better cancer (dreadful though it is), you may think, than Alzheimer's or motor neurone or some other disease you have hardly heard of but is no doubt lurking there somewhere in the shadows ready to pounce on you.

People are bound to notice the signs of senility in body and mind – the loss of capacities they did not know they had until they lost them: their tendency to tiredness; the worsening of their short-term memory and their ability to bring ideas into a pattern; their powers of concentration; their trembling hands; the weakening of this or that other gift – messages which spill over themselves when they have cancer or any other normally fatal illness. Even when perfectly healthy they cannot avoid noticing that others regard them as old. The unlucky old can be ghettoised early into the old people's homes which are a feature of the kind of nomad society industrial countries are becoming. Unlucky they may be, but perhaps not quite so much so as old and feeble people in more simple nomad societies who are left to die when their band moves on.

Here are some of the older people. First, Harold Allen, the gaunt ex-soldier, 75 when he died. In his six years in the army, which he enjoyed so much that he wanted to stay on as a professional soldier, he saw all manner of deaths. Death had been very close to him then and he could not be quite so afraid of it again as people who had not brushed so closely with it. 'It doesn't worry you,' he said, 'when you've seen all that.' He was emphatic that 'I'm not afraid of dying,' and he had to be believed. 'I shan't be a bit sorry to die, to see if there is an afterlife or if there is not one, so it is a great adventure.'

This did not mean that, in his unassertive way, he wanted to die. Although he was so ill that his life had been given up, he was quite clear that, if he was going to die, he did not want to die in a hospital, amongst nurses at least one of whom he regarded with fierce hostility. For him age was on the side of death, family on the side of life.

Walter Bliss was a good deal older.

Walter Bliss (94)

Cancer of glands and throat. Widower, living in Stepney, with one son, Eddie, living nearer to him than his two daughters. An ex-docker, who still conveys a sense of the powerful man he once was, he is at the time we see him confined by his swollen legs and feet to his home, indeed to one room within it – his kitchen. He sits there facing the front door of the flat with everything he needs no further away than arm's length – papers, letters, newspapers, coffee on the table, a timetable for his eye medication pinned to a board near enough for him to see. His walking frame is laced with wires so that if he does have to move around at all his stereo radio moves with him.

Despite his very restricted life, Walter had brought one precious asset with him from his past. As a docker and a member for most of his life of the same stable East London community, he had a 'reputation', a good reputation embodying the values held dear by a lot of people he knew. He had pride in himself, reinforced by the pride which other people had in him, and he still had it even though the community of which he had been such a stalwart member had almost disappeared. He knew who he was; he had a strong sense of identity and this, it seemed, enabled him to face death with courage. He was not going to let down his reputation in his own eyes or in anyone else's.

But he no longer had any strong wish to live. 'You can't deceive yourself about it. I'm 93.' And, more important, Walter felt much more alone since his wife died, in this like Arthur Jacobs, and as Alice Colyer felt about her husband. Her absence was Walter's constant regret.

I wish my wife would come back. I do. I talk to her. I'm a lonely old man. I wake up at night and think of her and cry myself to sleep.

Three or four years before we met, a daughter had died and while we knew him, a sister and a son-in-law. There was not much left to attach him to life.

Jack Dickson was the same in one important way – having a

'character' which had been well known to many people of his acquaintance.

Jack Dickson (77)

Colon cancer. Spitalfields. Widower. Of seven brothers, only he and another one in New Zealand are left. Of his five sisters, two survive and come to see him. He had worked for much of his life in a local vegetable market. He is a natural comic who tells stories to us and anyone who would listen, as a juggler would throw coloured balls into the air for the amazement of others.

Jack, known as Jimminy, had a large fund of such stories.

I like making people laugh. Everybody knows me. I'll tell you, I was walking along the market one day with a friend and he met a friend of his who didn't say hello. I said, 'Why don't you say hello to me?,' and he said, 'I don't know you.' I said, 'I'm Jimminy, everyone knows me, the Pope knows me.' 'Go on,' he said. 'Yes,' I said. 'You come to Italy with me and I'll show you.' So we eventually come to Italy and to the Vatican and I left my friend with an Italian friend and my friend said, 'How will I know it's the Pope?' Then two people came out on the balcony of the Vatican and my friend said, 'How do I know that's the Pope?' So he asked an Italian passing by, 'Antonio, is that the Pope up there?' 'I don't know,' said Antonio, 'but it's Jimminy standing next to him.'

He was certainly well known in the Spitalfields Vegetable Market where he'd worked as a tea-boy for the porters while at school, and then got a job there when he first left school. The market porters all belonged to three big families, the Filsons, the Langtons and the Barneys. Jimminy's mother was a Filson, Mrs Langton was a Filson. Seventy members of the three families were employed there, mostly fathers and sons. When fathers died, sons took over. Jimminy's mother had ten sons, Mrs L. twelve, Mrs B. fourteen. All the carts belonged to Jimminy's uncles, the Langtons. Jimminy had a horse and cart for delivering potatoes to fish and chip shops and eel and pie shops all over the East

End. His market was a market for everything. 'You could buy an elephant or a pin. Drivers would bring eggs and sell them among the porters. Others would bring shirts which they wasn't supposed to. It was all educational.' It was like going to the theatre every day, amicable, jokes all day long.

As with Walter, Jack's reputation was still almost a living presence for him, an alter ego, and it was this that was carrying him through a series of crises. The past was so vivid for him, so much more than the nowaday everyday that the past had eclipsed the present. He was living then rather than now. It was as if when he walked out into the street he would be greeted by hundreds of reassuring ghosts of the Filsons, the Langtons and the Barneys. Living alone, he was still not lonely: he had that past to inhabit.

The present was not so good. He had a great-niece who had recently taken him out in her car to one of the pubs he used to go to. She said, 'Some of your old pals want to see you.' There was a chap playing the piano. He turned and said, 'What are you doing, Jimminy?' and J. replied, 'I'm trying to breathe.' 'Oh,' he said, 'and I was going to ask you to sing.' He didn't want to go to a pub again after that. The past was more comforting and made him willing to accept death when it came without too much protest. The past brought him a sense of peace, especially when it crossed his mind that he might be rejoining the past in the future. Alice was quite explicit about accepting death.

Alice Colyer (80)

Colon cancer. Widow in Bethnal Green. One daughter, Sarah. A very small woman, bent over by arthritis, who leans heavily on her stick as she walks. A very private person, she shuts herself up in her spacious terraced house with only an abandoned unfriendly cat for company. She talks a lot to the cat, without response.

Alice did not dread death:

When I was your age, if anyone had asked, I'd have been terrified of dying but not now. As you grow older it becomes inevitable. I'm not afraid of dying, no, nor the manner of dying. I just don't think about it. It doesn't trouble me at all.

Alice was happy, despite her cancer and despite the uncommunicative cat. Her only real sadness was not having her husband with her. 'I'm not completely happy because I've not got my husband. We were lovely together.' But she had spirit enough to pack her bags and depart the hospital when the surgeon treated her discourteously (we come back to this incident in Chapter 5).

Arthur Jacobs also seemed untroubled by the prospect before him.

Arthur Jacobs (72)

Lung cancer. He is a sunny Jewish widower in Whitechapel, with a glint to his eye, and a lovely smile. He has three children by his first marriage and three by his second. Sitting under a picture embroidered by his second wife, he rolls and smokes the cigarettes which are presumably his downfall, something he learnt to do in the army and has never been able to give up since.

Arthur spoke in very much a matter-of-fact way about his funeral, as though he expected to be there.

Donald Knight said less about what was coming.

Donald Knight (74)

Cancer of the prostate. Married to Ivy, without children, but with siblings on both sides of the family. A thin man, with thinning hair, dark deep-set eyes which don't meet yours, and heavy glasses. Ivy, small and cheerful, says you can set your watch by the time Donald asks for his morning drink. Welcoming rather than resenting it, she had taught herself to be prompt.

At least Donald did not express any particular fears. He had always hated being alone. When his wife Ivy went to hospital for a gall bladder operation a few years previously, Donald had phoned his sister every day asking her to come round. He couldn't stand the flat without Ivy in it. Ivy and he had talked a lot about which one would go first. After his death Ivy told us she was quite glad it had turned out she had not been the first and that she had been there to look after him. Like almost all the other elderly people, Donald thought a great deal about the past and, in doing so, he was from different angles binding together into a whole the experience of a lifetime.

Amongst these older people, Dora Anstey (the widow who suffered from the cold) was the exception. Despite her age she was not the least tolerant of what was about to happen. She was resentful about it. Perhaps this was due to her having made a deep relationship with a man-friend not long before; she may have harboured the hope that she could still make up for some of the failings in previous relationships. Dora's attitude suggested to us that it is not age as such which softens the prospect of death but the effect which age has on people's spirits. Age can make it seem that nature is at work to bring on what is as inevitable for people as for cats, dogs, flies, wasps, elephants or any other living creature or living thing; but only if their spirit does not pull them away from that common ending. Speaking generally, one of the many benefits (to set against the disadvantages) of living well into old age was that death was easier to accept.

The younger

The others were somewhat younger. It is counter-intuitive for younger people to die before older, as though contrary to natural justice. Their general inclination was the opposite, to struggle against the onset of death (or, as it can also be thought of, the unseemly acceleration of ageing that dying implies) with all the vigour they could muster. They were not among the young who are supposed to be more ready to die, in war or adventure. The youngest of them was 39 and they were a bit more like other middle-aged and older people who have been described elsewhere.

Prosperity knits a man to the world. He feels that he is finding his place in it while really it is finding its place in him. His increasing reputation, his widening circle of acquaintances, his sense of importance, the growing pressure of absorbing and agreeable work build up a sense of being really at home on earth.[13]

There were exceptions amongst the younger of our people who were unlike the conventional picture of the young and not unwilling to die. Dermot, the Irish loner mentioned before, had an unusually miserable life, with no prospects of it improving. Poverty separated him from his family at an early age. While his sister remained at home, he was sent to an industrial boarding school when he was 7 and left when he was 14. The school was ruled by the lash of the Christian brothers who ran it. He was taught a trade, how to make boots, but was not able to use it. Unfortunate from the start of his life, there seemed to be nothing much on this earth that was worth striving for.

Derek Wood was more difficult to fathom.

Derek Wood

In his early fifties with lung cancer in a house in Newham, he is the secretary of a religious trust, who was working normally until a month before we met him. Divorced, with children he is estranged from. A good man saddened by a sad life. He wears a suit and waistcoat and his manner of speaking is unusually courteous and formal even when talking about everyday things.

Derek had been living on his own. When he got ill he struck up a fulfilling relationship and lived with a Mrs Litten. She was a 'mothering type' and almost seemed to welcome his cancer because it gave her the opportunity to take on this role and him the opportunity to benefit from it. But through it all was a strong sense of resigned melancholy about him, as though his time was short and he would soon be catapulted forth onto the next stage of his journey. Like Dermot, he believed in an afterlife.

Janet Rahman also believed in an afterlife.

Janet Rahman (46)

Breast cancer. Hackney. Married with two daughters to a Muslim husband who also has a Muslim co-wife. A small woman with sad eyes whose grey hair makes her look older than her 46 years. Her husband is a strong-looking man on shiftwork who loves field hockey and avidly follows the fortunes of the Pakistan team.

Janet was in an upstairs room where she was to quite a large extent left alone. She was liable to 'panic attacks'.[14] There was not much to hold her to life. She was relieved that her Muslim husband was going to allow her daughter to marry whomever her daughter liked, instead of whom he liked. This was her last deeply felt wish. She felt calmer when it was granted.

The others wanted strongly to survive but expressed it in different ways. Carol Taylor, the attractive divorcee, was certainly not willing. Insofar as she struggled against death, she did so (like Jennifer Barnes) by denial of her plight, in this bearing out the importance given to denial by Dr Kubler-Ross. She repeatedly insisted she would recover and repeatedly managed to twist the information she was given so that it could support her show of optimism. To begin with, she was slow to do anything about the lump she could feel in her breast. She hoped it would go away.

> My hair was falling out, my teeth falling out. I'd lost weight but I'd still not realised.

She did not go to her GP for six months after her first serious symptoms appeared. With hindsight, she recognised that this had been a mistake, but she still got the reassurance she wanted from him. She continually reported what doctors said in a way that was favourable to her; but we never had the sense that they could have actually said what she said they said.

> He said if they had caught the breast in time it would have been fine but it will have taken five to ten years off my life. I asked him how long am I going to have. He said 'as long as you want'. I wanted to know if this would bring my life expectancy from 60 to 55. He said 'as long as you are sensible and take the treatment you will survive'.

After she had finally consulted doctors she had a lumpectomy – this was five years before we saw her – but did not think it could be serious enough to justify radiotherapy thereafter. She feared its effects. But a year later she had her breast removed and followed this with the radiotherapy she had refused before. She shook off the dust of that ward as though (despite it) she must now be cured for good; to demonstrate the cure, with a display of the utmost energy she decorated her flat from top to bottom, and returned to work for two years in her full-time job in her old occupation as a confidential secretary.

Her brother and sister had both had cancer before her. Her brother had taken it particularly hard.

> My brother broke down and wouldn't speak to anyone for six weeks. I couldn't let it do that to me. There are lots of people living with cancer and they will live, and live a long life. It's not going to kill you all the time. It will be uncomfortable etc. and there'll be some suffering. You have to get used to it.

Her mother looked after her and her daughter did not, or not to the same extent. Fearing, sensibly, that she was misremembering what doctors said, she got into the habit of taking her mother with her on all her hospital visits. But her mother did not manage any better than she did. Her mother said about the consultations with doctors: 'It's so quick and everything. They're talking to you and not talking to you.'

Later on came the relapse and, although the signs were as obvious as before, she did nothing about it for quite some time. She noticed she could not move her little finger, then her right hand, then her right arm, and then she had a fit. After that she submitted to the hospital once more, and this time to the chemotherapy she had kept clear of until then. She was frightened by the ward she was in.

> It frightens me so much, people calling out at night, drips, dying, knowing the majority were terminal. I didn't feel I was in a ward where I'm normal. I didn't associate myself with that level of treatment.

Her appearance began to change; she did her best to cover it up. She still described it as a phase, after which she would get better. She was anxious to keep her friends away lest they were shocked by the alteration in her looks and confirm by the horror in their eyes that she was not getting better, at least for the time being. She prided herself on keeping things going. 'I still want to go to the gym for weight training and aerobics. I can't at the moment while my hand's like this but it's so much better after only a fortnight.' She never spoke about the future she had lost. She did not believe she had lost it. But she did not get better.

Carol's method of holding off the disease was to ignore its seriousness. Her spirit was certainly engaged but not in such a way that she was open with herself. She had had many losses in her life, in her family of origin as well as in her family of marriage, and these losses may have made it near impossible to face realistically another, of herself. Her fear of her life being shortened was so great that she brought about what she feared, shortening it by ensuring that at different phases of the illness it was not 'caught in time'.

Along with her denial went a kind of acceptance of her situation, coupled with a religious attitude to it.

Having spoken with a priest recently in the hospital, he gave me a strength and comfort that I didn't realise I needed. The peace and tranquillity of the Church means that you can sit and think there where you can't anywhere else. I've felt better and calmer since I've spoken to the priest.

I still have the peace I got when I spoke with the priest at the hospital. Now, I pray more than I ever did. I've got a rosary upstairs and look at it every single night . . . it helps to calm me down.

The priest was very calming, peaceful. I felt as if I was actually being helped by God. I can still see his face and hear his voice. I never thought that I would need the spiritual support that I have done but when the chips are down you do need that little bit extra. If the time is up, I've got to know there is something up there waiting. It helps to know there is something beyond . . . something that makes it worthwhile . . . that it's not all been in vain.

Fighting spirit

Another two, Kenneth Chandler (67) and Julia Searle (54), had a more straightforward fighting spirit. As we have said before, Kenneth had been in and out of hospital. When cancer of the bladder was diagnosed, he was not operated on again: it was thought his heart (and his lungs which had also been affected) would not stand up to it. Instead, he had intensive radiotherapy in 1987, followed by chemotherapy, and a year later further chemotherapy. He passed blood frequently. He had pneumonia. His breathing was very poor. After such a catalogue of misfortune, Kenneth could have been more than forgiven if he had lost some of his zest for life. This he most emphatically had not.

In his sixth year after the first cancer diagnosis he had one in a long series of scares when he thought he had a secondary in his stomach. He had again lost a lot of weight. The Home Care doctor had been called and given him the 'thorough examination' so many patients crave for: he said that only a deep scan could tell more but he could find no visual evidence of a secondary cancer. Bucked by this, Kenneth immediately started to plan a trip. His older brother had emphysema and his younger brother had offered to take this brother (not Kenneth), and his new mobile oxygen carrier, on a trip to a Marks & Spencer store in Berkshire, this being near where their mother had taken the whole family from the Isle of Dogs in the general evacuation at the beginning of the war. Kenneth said to his older brother, 'Why not me as well?', and he was going to ask if he also could have a mobile oxygen carrier so that he would be at no disadvantage on this daring journey.

Julia Searle was like Carol in one vital respect. She had the same kind of cancer.

Julia Searle (54)

Breast and other cancers. Single. Once a radiographer, she is a cheerful, sardonic, intelligent person who can wring pleasure out of the most unlikely and terrible events. While she talks, her strong hands with their finely manicured nails hold out, as if for admiration, the equally long thin cigarettes she smokes to the end of her illness. A Burmese cat lies in front of the gas fire in her stylishly furnished flat in Hackney.

Julia had, as we noticed earlier in this chapter, survived for many years after she first had breast cancer. No doubt the longer people survive, the more confident they are liable to feel that they will go on defeating death. They may think that, if dying can be slowed down enough, their trajectory will eventually join that of the normal slow decline of normal healthy people.

In most other ways Julia was very different from Carol. She did not have an ordinary family around her. Her mother and father were a long way off and not well and she seldom saw either them or an only brother who was so extremely busy with his job that he hardly ever had time to see her, even when she was desperately ill. She also had what Carol did not have, faithful friends including one, Maria, not in a lesbian relationship but closer to her, and more attentive, more helpful, more loving, than almost any sister or daughter could ever be. Although she lived alone apart from her beloved cat, Hermione, she also had the greatest affection for her flat; there she was in complete control of what little happened and there she had the precious objects she had collected over a lifetime, the china, the glass vases and the pictures. But it was not her family, or lack of it, or her home, which could explain the spirit which had carried her through the purgatory of thirteen years since the first diagnosis of breast cancer and then a cancerous tumour in her arm, and rheumatoid arthritis, and kidney cancer, and multiple hernias, and cancer of the bone marrow.

Her spirit was shown by her wish for treatment far beyond the point where most people would give up in despair or resignation. She held on tightest in her last stages, when the cancer had so far eaten away her bone that her spine was threatening to collapse. She had a stainless steel halo fitted round her head with bars that fixed into a plaster cast gripping her shoulders and the upper part of her body. The halo around her head was screwed into her scalp at four points. While she was in the Royal Marsden (a specialist cancer hospital) she asked to see one of us. Here is part of the note made on the visit:

She is sitting up in a chair looking out from under the halo. Her head is completely rigid. She cannot move it from side to side by as much as a centimetre. Only her eyes can move but two screws going into her skull are directly above each eye so that her vision is partly obscured. The plaster cast is biting into her shoulder. She asks me to sit on the bed directly in front of her so that she can see me. She can move her hands and manage to light one of her long brown cigarettes, looking as unswervingly at me as before. Was the traffic bad on the way? she asks.

The halo was not enough by itself and when there was the prospect of another operation in an orthopaedic hospital (where the staff were not used to cancer patients and didn't understand the drugs for controlling cancer pain) to put in plates and wires to strengthen her spine, she jumped at it with enthusiasm and did everything she could to persuade the surgeon to undertake it, although the chances of success were slim. If against all the odds it succeeded, she thought she might have as long as another year to live. The operation took seven hours.

A hole had to be made in her neck for this operation and a week or so later the wound opened up with a little click. She was in agony. There was a chance, again eagerly seized, of yet another operation to take flesh from another part of her body to patch up the hole. The attempt failed, as it did in a further operation for the same purpose.

She said she did not want a church service but a member of the clergy to conduct a ceremony around her grave. Meanwhile, she was as delighted as ever to return home.

Death be not proud, though some have called thee
Mighty and dreadful, for thou art not so.[15]

What accounted for her remarkable spirit which kept her going and kept her cheerful almost all the time, while always being rooted in a realistic appreciation of her plight? We would only mention three other facts about her which struck us, her links with the medical professions, her sense of humour and her self-respect.

1 When she was struck down she had been a radiologist in an NHS hospital. Having to work many years with out-of-date x-ray equipment which the hospital could not afford to replace may have been one of the precipitators of her cancer. This meant she already knew a good deal about it and the possible treatments. She knew, too, about the rather rapid progress being made in developing them and this could strengthen the hope that if only she could hold on.... She could join in the discussions with her doctors – they could keep no secrets from her – almost as though she was one of them. She appreci-

ated them; they appreciated her, especially her courage and her concern for other people. They were the fraternity she felt she belonged to.

2 Her sense of humour never seemed to desert her. Very few kinds of authority are immune to that barb, and it was almost as if she was intent upon testing whether death too could be faced down. She started off her many long conversations with us by explaining, with a sparkle in her eye, that she was terminal, not terminal terminal, and although it was a joke it also expressed her attitude. It was going to take a lot to turn her into a terminal terminal. She went through a religious experience (not sustained at all afterwards) in the earlier stages of her illness and saw a good deal of priests. Religion amused her as well. On one of her hospital stays

> the priest came by one day. We were chatting away and then suddenly his hand was firmly on my knee. Let us pray he said. For what? I thought, then back we were talking as if nothing had happened.

She had a stay in a hospice but was terrified lest, in accord with their mission, they would not resuscitate her. The night staff might not realise she was not terminal terminal. She asked the doctor to put on her notes 'This patient is to be resuscitated', extracting some wry amusement from her slight guying of the hospice.

3 She was mortified by the awful changes in her looks and by her feeble efforts with her trembling hands to get make-up on to her face in the right places before she went to out-patients. But beneath the skin and behind her wracked body she retained a steady sense of herself throughout it all. She kept that intact, safe from any knife. It was a kind of pride but not an immodest one. Her sense of identity being so strong, she was always interested in other people. In her last days she could not walk. Any weakness in her legs would show her the paralysis was starting again. Her right arm was weaker. We noted:

> She can't hold a spoon. It could be the beginning of a more general paralysis. She has two electrodes in her arm shooting a small current through in an attempt to outmanoeuvre the pain and two morphine syringes, one in her arm and one in her leg. One of the home nurses asked her how she could

stay so cheerful. She said, 'I don't feel cheerful'. The nurse said, 'yes but you are'.

Whether a fighting spirit makes final death any easier or more difficult we do not know, and even those who are very close at the end can do no more than guess. But during the period which leads up to it, such a spirit certainly does give something to live for. To hold off death can be an achievement almost beyond compare.

* * *

In this chapter we have introduced the patients who were our subjects and our partners, mentioning the inescapables (above all the cancer itself) which they could do so little about, and the free variables – the degrees to which they could express their individuality, and draw on their own capacities, even in such an extremity. What stands out is the significance of people's spirit – this for want of a better word for a quality that belongs to a whole personality and the whole reaction of that personality to adversity. Of its manifestations we have been able to do no more than catch a glimpse. But that the consequences to the individual are immense we have no doubt.

Chapter 3

The battle for independence

All our people had to cope with the mental distress which 'may be perhaps the most intractable pain of all'.[1] They had to give up their future.[2] They did not suddenly realise, as if seeing the figure of death knocking at their front door, that they who had been going to live for ever were now about to die. They had exchanged one uncertainty for another, but it was far from an exchange of like for like. The new uncertainty was not about the timing of a death so far off that it did not have to be pondered, but about a death so near that worry about the timing could not be avoided. They had given up the happy uncertainty of the healthy for the nagging uncertainty of the very ill, which has sometimes been regarded as being even worse than certainty, though not, we think, by many people who are themselves dying. As a committed proponent of a quick death, Inglis said:

> The fact that the time between diagnosis and death may vary from weeks to years has tended only to add to cancer's ill-repute, much as a judicial death sentence is harder to bear if the condemned man does not know the date of his execution.[3]

Some people – hypochondriacs of one degree or another – fear they are to die when they contract any illness at all, even a bout of 'flu; as long as they feel worse day by day, they can at once precipitate themselves down a private chute into the crematorium. But most illnesses yield no such omen. They are not considered as serious as that. They are illnesses from which people get better, and once they turn the corner (as the saying goes), they find it the easiest and most agreeable thing in the world to extrapolate themselves back into their seat in the pub, conviviality all round them; or back, potency abounding, behind the steering wheel of the car which has been waiting so faithfully outside their house for them to get better.

The illnesses of our people were not like that. They were taken so seriously by general practitioners that people suddenly stopped being people and became patients under someone else's orders. It was not for nothing that people customarily spoke of being 'under' – 'I am under the doctor' – even as one speaks of being put 'under' an anaesthetic. They could cease overnight to be a person – or at any rate the same person – when they were consigned to wait their turn in giant buildings (the largest buildings many people ever go into) full of bustling strangers in white coats who, though strangers, may well have a terrifying power of clairvoyance about their future. So clear did it become that from such an illness there might be no recovery that procrastination about death could no longer be preserved quite intact; it had to be replaced by the much more disturbing possibility of the truth.

The patients were then liable to envy people with ordinary illnesses almost more than quite healthy people; one of their dearest wishes was to have a simple, ordinary, reassuring sort of illness as so often in the past. Dora Anstey, the frail widow who always felt cold, said, 'I just want someone to take this off my shoulders and tell me it's going to be alright and give me some medicine and I'll get better. I know that it can't be done but that's what I want.' Jennifer Barnes, the Afro-Caribbean nurse, liked to think she was just out of sorts. She noticed, 'When people are just normally ill, nothing really bothers them because they know they are going to get better. Deep down I'm thinking all the time since last weekend I just feel out of sorts.' Julia Searle, the former radiographer, said in the orthopaedic hospital where she went that the other patients in for operations were not really ill. 'They just have a technical hitch which will soon be put right.' She wished she too had a technical hitch. Some people could fool themselves some of the time; since none could fool themselves all the time, the fear was also that the illness could be incurable, not in the way that many diseases like asthma or diabetes are incurable and kept under control, but both incurable and soon to take control.

Messages from within

The intimations of mortality came not just from the doctors
(when and if they spoke up) but from the alarming changes
within the patients themselves. When people did what one doctor
said they should do, listen to their bodies, what they heard was
not reassuring. The body which had been the kind friend for so
long, and given so much pleasure, had turned into a stranger,
even an enemy, and was making itself felt almost as though it
was an alien creature, bringing on an awareness of capacities they
did not know they had until they lost them. Instead of being one
body they were two, a body which was afflicted and a mind
looking on. They were made aware by the complaint coming
from within of how much they had taken for granted. The physical
deterioration could not be denied, and the decline pointed to
only one future, none at all. Any sharp change, even an improvement (like a promotion), can bring on a sense of loss. 'Old
patterns of thought and activity must be given up and fresh
ones developed ... the transition involves giving up one set of
assumptions about the world and establishing another; grief is
the inevitable consequence.'4 But it is much worse when the
change is not at all an improvement but a disaster.

They had to recognise they were not as strong as they had
been; and they were going to be still less so unless, with or
without the aid of medical science, they were to have a reprieve.
The decline, and the rate of decline, constituted linear time paths
of a most fundamental sort. It stared people in the face – sometimes literally, as when Julia, after taking steroids, looked in her
mirror.

It was a terrible shock when I first saw my face in the mirror. It
was all orangey colour, with thick black hair hanging around it.

Cancer unfolds at different rates according to its type and the
effectiveness of the treatment designed to slow it down. Usually,
it is no runaway decline. The unfolding is gradual even for those
with a relatively fast growth, and the onset of disability likewise.
To begin with, it may hardly be noticed; and one of the surprises
for several people was that they could apparently (according to
their doctors) be so ill when they had no (or little) pain.

Several people were able to go on working at their jobs for
months or years after the onset. But then came the time when

they could no longer carry on. They lost their jobs and their incomes – it was premature retirement for those who had not already retired – and, from then on, one loss succeeded another. 'That hurt,' said Jennifer, 'taking the future away from me. I had this job option of retiring at 60 or 65 and the illness has just taken it away.' 'It is difficult coming to terms with not being needed,' said Julia when she felt it was not fair on her colleagues to stick at her work any longer. It was worse later on when an occupational therapist advised special fitments around her loo and other safety measures. It suddenly struck her. 'I'm being treated as a disabled person and not expected to get well again.'

But even in their new situation, as we try to show in this chapter, they were by no means helpless. They could maintain and make use of their independence as human beings. Given the nature of our culture, and the significance attached to being in control, the issue became one of critical importance in the illness. The observation that great emergencies show us how much greater our vital resources are than we had supposed was borne out again and again, as also the other observation that 'an event which may be a crisis for one person can be a moment of unperplexing opportunity for another'.[5]

Loss of mobility

Early on in the illness, mobility was little impaired except when recovering from operations and other drastic treatments. People could go on driving until a ban was decreed. This was as much a watershed as for old people forced to give up when they recognise (or others recognise for them) that they are getting slower on the brakes than they were, less accurate in their steering, less sure in their judgement about anything. Kenneth Chandler, the man with the carriage of a lightweight boxer, was told at the hospital: ' "In my opinion I don't think you should drive." That flipped me down a bit.' He gave his car to one of his daughters. Until absolutely compelled to, Carol Taylor, the attractive divorcee, did not take the advice she was given.

The hospital said I shouldn't be driving but if I can't drive a car I can't go out. I go to the hospital by car and drive myself – I've not told them. But driving is the one thing I can still do and enjoy.

After they could no longer drive, several people could still take short walks out of the house. Walter, the former docker, could manage it in the right season. 'It's a little better in the summertime because I can't walk against this wind.' Some could pace themselves by measuring the distances they could manage, hoping each day to manage a few steps more in the hope that such firm objective measurement would convince them they were actually improving. Harold, the once tall soldier, was at one stage highly satisfied. 'I can walk from here to the corner opposite the park. Yesterday I managed to get round the bend in the road.' Clinging to Lilian's arm, he might have added. Reading a book and maintaining concentration for half an hour or so could also be an achievement. Derek, the courteous divorcee, was very positive about the progress he was making:

> There's gradual improvement all through. I'm eating much better. My weight has begun to climb again. Things are beginning gradually to improve for which I'm grateful. I've been out most days to and fro from the hospital and the doctor, and most days I've taken a walk around or go to the pub. I walk 200 yards and in the public house there I'll have a quiet drink with two or three friends.

A few days later Derek was dead.

As people's range was further cut down, they could not manage stairs and were confined to the span of a room or two on one level. But they still had the vital freedom of being able to move around the room and out of it to the bathroom, even if, after a couple of steps, breathlessness made them stand still and hold on to a cupboard or a door to rest. Donald, who liked promptness, had once been a keen football player, and he could still play little games. When he was feeling good he might suddenly get up from his chair and (as his wife, Ivy, put it) 'take these little walks into the kitchen to see what's going on in there'. What was going on was that Ivy was sitting there.

> I get so tired just sitting here.   (Donald)
>
> Yes, I look up and there he is coming to see what he can find.   (Ivy)

Donald could not bath himself on his own.

We managed a bath this week. Each time it's a little more difficult. (Ivy)

I nearly toppled over. (Donald)

Yes, next time we'll use the top seat and I'll get one of those little showers to put on the taps so that I can keep warm water going over Don's body. (Ivy)

I can't have a good soak now. That's what I really used to like. (Donald)

Even limited mobility was very precious. When he got out of bed, Harold wobbled 'like a newborn calf'. But if he managed to keep his balance he could slowly shave himself and brush his teeth before taking a long rest to recover from his exhausting exertions. Donald was very slow too. One of his first actions was to go to the lavatory. 'I sit there for a long time and it presses on the nerve in my left leg and I get a lot of pain.' After that he rested for 15 minutes before returning to the bathroom to shave, which took him half an hour. He would then sleep or pretend to sleep until 11 a.m. when, according to Ivy, 'He'll open one eye and say it's Bovril time.'

Those who had problems with their balance were, like Donald, afraid they would topple right over. This happened to Dora. 'I was alright before the fall,' she said. A few months before, Alice Colyer, the small woman bent over with arthritis, had fallen, on the way to church. 'I could have cried with vexation. I felt so conspicuous.' At least she was not seriously hurt. Others when they fell could hear the crunching sound of a bone breaking. A broken limb could mean hospital again and all the terrible things that could happen there.

Derek's fear was that in a dizzy spell he would lean too hard on the banisters and be found dead at the bottom of the stairs. The fear of falling was general, but hardly less so was distaste for the means by which it might be prevented – the walking frame and the wheelchair. Kenneth held out tenaciously against being put in a wheelchair when he went to the hospital and the same at home. 'A wheelchair would make me feel an invalid and I'm not an invalid.' He would rather be walking wounded than not walking. He had to admit though, as he lost strength, that it was sometimes not so unpleasant.

They took me to Marks & Spencer in Reading. It's a vast

store and when we got there the supervisor came up with a wheelchair. My sisters had phoned ahead and arranged it. Oh, it was a beautiful wheelchair.

Ability to move about – even the minimal but crucial degree necessary to get from their regular station in an armchair to the other station on the lavatory or to a telephone to ask for help – was essential to the maintenance of some independence. Without it, control over themselves in their little bit of space was almost gone. To have to be lifted on to a commode or lavatory and held there was getting on for the ultimate in indignity, complete double incontinence being one condition worse. The loss of the capacity to take a few steps was also enough to make it nearly impossible to stay at home. The patient could be too heavy for one person to lift on to his feet.

With this as the prospect, the patients had to use whatever remained of their independence to maintain their independence, and, however much of an immense effort it took, struggle to walk. If one did not walk, one would soon not be able to. Use it or lose it. Dermot Donoghue, the quiet Irishman, said, 'You must keep your legs going, or that's it, isn't it?' Julia Searle spent long hours whenever she was getting near to discharge from a hospital or hospice practising walking. On one occasion a friend brought her some trainers for her painful dragging up and down the corridor. When you see elderly people in the street with every step an effort you know why they are doing it.

Immobility could add to the other losses – loss of friends, loss of the use of an arm or a hand, loss of the ability to move around even within the confines of a room, loss of the power of concentration, loss of confidence in what your body could take, loss of control over your bowels, and a generalised fear about which function was to be impaired next. For Harold and his wife, 'We meet it in stages as it goes along', and 'we' did not give in at all easily. Walter Bliss used once to box for the army. Now he had lost weight, from 13 stones down to 6. 'I'm not a man, not a man.' But he often tried to show he had not lost all his strength. Arthur Jacobs lost height as well as weight but there were still many things he could do. Loss of appetite was gradual too. It was like this with personal interests, except that it was more difficult to force them into life when they were vanishing. Jack said: 'I used to go potty when snooker and cricket were on the telly. Now I've got no more interest.' The most he could do was to keep up with his weekly football coupons.

Often the decline was not steady. It was punctuated by hospital appointments which could be frequent at times of crisis – 'I've got more appointments than the Queen'. At the level of fantasy the awful things that could happen had been well-rehearsed beforehand. The visits were dreaded because at this local temple of judgement they had to give an account of themselves to the other human being who had taken so much of their lives under his or her control. If found wanting, there would be some new complication that could accelerate the decline.

But it was not always like that. A hospital visit could also bring hope of some betterment. The main treatments – surgery, radiotherapy and chemotherapy – were given there and, while they were all liable to be unpleasant, particularly in their side effects, they were also often followed by a remission which allowed people to resume some of their old activities. When people were admitted as in-patients, they had, of course, to con- form to the rigid institutional cycles of the hospital and surrender their own more idiosyncratic ones to the general rule. But if all went well with their stay or with their outpatient treatment, it could be (as one of them put it) like a 'rebirth' when it was over. It could seem like a miracle to people who feared they would die in hospital; and once they had got over the first shock of having to take more responsibility for themselves again and assumed the burdens of freedom, the living room at home, with its many reminders and reassurance of ordinary life, could seem a little heaven to return to, especially when one might soon be able to move around it. It was at home that one could be independent and amongst other things use the telephone to invite people to visit or to keep them away in a manner not possible in hospital. In-patients are at the disposal of their friends and at the mercy of their enemies.

This is not from a social point of view to decry the value of hospital. There they could meet fellow-patients, including ones met before, perhaps as an in-patient. A ward (like a more ordinary battlefield) can be a hot-house for friendships, bringing them into flower more quickly than in everyday life. People who have been on a ward together form a clannish group for mutual support and it becomes a pleasure to see one of them again on a later visit. Adversity produces solidarity. 'In any hospital,' said

Julia, 'people become very friendly. It's a very intimate relationship. It never happens in ordinary life – fetching bedpans, taking
out your false teeth. People band together against doctors and
nurses. You all support anyone who's been told something nasty.'
People worse off than you can also give a strange sense of comfort. You have been so sorry for yourself, but now there are all
these others.

> Being there made me realise the severity of my illness but I
> felt a fraud because their level of suffering was much greater
> than mine.   (Carol)

> There are lots of other patients around. That's good for you
> because there'll always be one patient worse off than you.
> (Julia)

Kenneth had been through more than most of the other patients;
he had survived and was cheerful about it – a veteran. Twice
people had asked him in hospital to talk to relatives about their
cancer. 'You don't look as if you've got cancer. I wish you'd
speak to my brother-in-law.' 'It's mind over matter, love.'

They could also just exchange information with each other. Dr
Clement-Jones, a cancer patient as well as doctor and, before she
died, the founder of BACUP (the British Association of Cancer
United Patients), saw this exchange as an important addition to
anything people got from their doctors.

> I finally met a fellow young patient with ovarian cancer. We
> shared our experiences.... Through this... I realised that
> other patients could give me something unique which I could
> not obtain from my doctors or nurses, however caring.
>
> I realised that there were two levels of information... one
> on a medical professional level and the other drawing on my
> experience as a 'veteran' patient who had knowledge that only
> someone who has 'been there' has. It became clear that the
> doctors and nurses had provided me only with the first level
> of information. The personal experience was unique to patients
> and their families and friends. This vast wealth of experience
> I felt was not being tapped effectively.... The concept of
> BACUP has evolved from the need to combine the two levels
> of information I describe – medical and experiential.[6]

So supportive to each other are these informal groups of patients who have been in hospital together that it could be one of the functions of hospital administrators to keep them together by giving them out-patient appointments on the same day unless there is good reason not to. They could amongst other things be put in touch with the self-help bodies like CANCER LINK, BACUP and CYANO (Cancer You Are Not Alone). Medicine could build, and build on, patient solidarity. If such miniature groups proved therapeutic as well as comforting, it could make isolated private rooms in hospital a lot less desirable.

The struggle for independence

Although treatment could slow things down and other patients could be a comfort, at the stage the disease had reached in our people, decline there had been and more decline there was likely to be. How was it to be dealt with other than by the kind of denial expressed by Carol, who twisted the information given to her by doctors so that it always seemed optimistic? If you did not close your eyes to what was happening to you, how were you to avoid being overwhelmed by depression?

The most general answer seemed to be that you should (1) prepare for the worst and (2) let your spirits rise when the worst does not happen. The first maxim is implicit in the value placed on openness which is more fully dealt with in Chapter 5. Openness means that the information possessed by doctors should not be concealed from patients (unless the patients want it to be); and the information is not only that someone has cancer but about its likely course of development and the treatments worth considering. Only if patients have that sort of information will they retain enough of their independence for the key decisions about whether to have this or that sort of treatment to be theirs rather than the doctors', or the doctors' alone. The doctors say what is on offer, and give their advice; the patients decide whether to accept the offer. People can also prepare in their minds for what is likely to happen. This can take the form of rehearsals even for small emergencies. Derek said:

> I'm afraid of having an attack of breathlessness. It can happen at any time. I have an immediate response. I take out my teeth.

It can even involve preparation for death itself. Several studies

have suggested that bereavement is eased a little if the survivors have ample time to cushion themselves against the shock.[7]
We will be referring to them again in Chapter 7. It would be
surprising if there was not something of the same benefit for
people anticipating their own death.

Harold said his goodbyes in hospital and also told people what
he 'expected' of them in terms of family support and cohesion.
He made sure of his wife's physical security and put his mind at
rest about her financial situation. He gave away certain treasured
items to relatives who would benefit from them, books to one of
his sons and his brushes and polishes to a grandson training in
french polishing, his old craft.

Julia sought to re-unite her family, that is her brother with her
mother in particular, and achieved this in part by bringing them
to speaking terms with each other. She made provision for the
future of her cat, Hermione. She made a detailed will – for
example, her opal ring to go to her mother and then to Maria
on her mother's death.

Mrs Champion moved in to look after Carol and her daughter,
Diane, as we said in Chapter 2. The will that Carol made provided
for the status quo to continue, through her mother living with
and continuing to care for Diane. But Carol's sister, Elaine, was
to be trustee for her daughter until she came of age. As it turned
out, Carol did not have the assets which she said should go to
her mother. In this respect her preparation for death was more
a matter of form than content.

Kenneth made a better job of it. He simplified his life by
immediately giving away any money that came his way. He felt
secure in the warmth of his family and was worried only about
grandson Philip's affection.

The first half of the maxim – preparing for the worst – is the
context in which the second can operate. The contentment or
discontent, the sadness or joy, which people feel, is largely the
consequence of comparing actuality with expectation. No human
being can avoid having expectations of the future, and of many
different futures with hundreds of different time-spans to them –
the next hour, the next day, the next week, the next month
and the next year, and many other intervals which are not tied
into the general Western chronology which has been constructed
since Julius Caesar gave his name to July and devised the Julian
Calendar. Expectations usually have unstated probabilities put on

them, and a diagnosis of cancer generates a new expectation of death which is no less pressing because it may not be immediately fulfilled. The expectations matter because they are the ground for making decisions about the future and because they constantly affect people's state of mind, people's moods, in the present. People employ them to produce greater stability for themselves than they would have otherwise – exaggerating how grim things are going to be so that the actuality when it comes is not so bad, and expecting good things to turn out a bit less well in practice. For people who are gravely ill, part of the value of preparing for the worst is that an outcome which is not as bad as the worst can be an occasion for a little rejoicing. The trick seems to be not to bury the worst and substitute fantasy for it but to allow the favourable to lift one's spirits as one contemplates the short-term future in which there may be an improvement – to be altogether flexible in the way expectations are formed and responded to. Just as the gloomy expectation of a long-term future is bound to colour one's view of the short term, so is a hopeful expectation of a short-term future bound to colour one's view of the longer term. On a day when one feels good one does not only feel good about that particular day.

The case for independence – for autonomy, freedom, liberty, for maintaining control, whatever words are used – is not just the familiar general case that is made in an individualistic society; it has a particular relevance for people who are seriously ill, or those whose independence is under threat from infirmity or age. Independence is always threatened by other people who, as experts, think they know better than those over whom their expertise gives them power. Doctors are particularly prone to infantilise their patients: they know so much more about our physical bodies than we do ourselves. But a doctor tempted to cut into people's minds as he can cut into their brains with his laser is committing a sin: he is depriving people of their humanity. He is taking away not just the power to take decisions but threatening to close out the brilliance with which the mind makes and remakes expectations in such a way that life remains worth living, and may be prolonged as well.[8] Julia thought that when she tidied her flat she was doing more than that.

You can only really fight if you are in control of your life; if not your immune system suffers.

Cancer greatly reduces freedom. What remains is all the more precious.

In this we are very much in agreement with Professor Wilkes, a doctor who has specialised in terminal care.

> We are at last beginning to realise that part of the art of medicine is not to prolong life but independence, for as long and as comfortably as possible.[9]

His view is not yet widely shared. Ordinary treatments aside, doctors have not yet given much attention to the art of prolonging independence and, with it, the morale of their patients. It is not yet thought to be a prime function of medicine to arouse and strengthen the will to live, to organise and to compensate for what has been lost. Our patients had to shift for themselves and maintain some control to prevent themselves from being over-come by their lack of a future. They wanted to do as much for themselves, and for others, as they possibly could, and they wanted to be given the chance to construct their own futures in a manner which was peculiarly their own. They needed carers, all the more as the illness progressed, but carers who would support them in their wish to help themselves as well as be helped.

What did this mean in practice? People employed two strategies in order to maintain their control:

1 took it day-by-day and on each day did as much as possible for themselves;
2 planned for limited but attainable goals.

The day-by-day

Several people did not quite follow the Bible: 'Take no thought for your life, what ye shall eat, or what ye shall drink; nor yet for your body, what ye shall put on. Is not the life more than meat, and the body than raiment?' (Matthew 6: 25). 'Take therefore no thought for the morrow: for the morrow shall take thought for the things of itself' (Matthew 6: 34). They did not want to exclude tomorrow completely. But they wanted to focus more sharply on the present. Janet, the co-wife, said the proper way to behave for people like her was to 'take each day as it comes and each day is precious to you'; Donald that 'we take it day by day'; and

Janet again that 'With God's help I say my prayers usually before I go to bed, thankful for the day I've had and hoping that I'll have a good day tomorrow.' Julia broadened the same thought to include, in with the 'us' of the terminally ill who are moving towards death at such a smart pace, the comity of all, the 'us' of humanity who think we are moving more slowly to the same destination. She said, 'Tomorrow is promised to none of us.' She went on to say, 'I have had to concentrate my thoughts on the day I am living. I have always been fighting for that one day and I haven't had time to think about my life as a whole.' People tried to make the scarcity of time work to their advantage, appreciating each day all the more because there were so few left.

When they succeeded, there was a narrowing down of time which fitted quite well with the narrowing down of space as they lost mobility. When we saw them, most had taken up their stations in the living rooms where they spent most if not all of their time. The living rooms were where they would choose to die, if they had their choice. This could be a perfectly good arrangement, even if the bed and sometimes a hoist or commode and other fitments made the living room look like a sickroom. Almost the only complaint was from people who regretted that the room in which they had settled was not on the ground floor with access to a little garden or yard where they might sometimes, if they could get so far, sun themselves and look at the flowers or the trees. 'I wish the flat were downstairs,' said Donald, 'so I could toddle into the garden.' This despite his general judgement that upstairs he had 'a really comfortable and cosy little room'. Julia rued the day when she had turned down a ground floor flat for one on the first floor. Although she loved going out it was liable to be ruined by the fear of having to heave herself up the stairs when she returned.

> Each day I think of something that I want to watch on TV or listen to on the radio and I concentrate on that.

By such means she tried to keep her thoughts on today and off tomorrow. She planned her day so that while she did one thing she also did another – say, listening to music *and* stroking her cat – and then there wouldn't be so much room left over in her mind for thinking dark thoughts. Kenneth, in similar vein, said that:

My greatest pleasure now, and I relish it every day, is just being alive. I think people take everyday things for granted. I treasure them.

Living for the day meant listening on the radio to the day's weather forecast. It meant taking part in, and being reassured by, many of the cycles within the day which are the same for anyone, healthy or ill, and which were the same as those they had followed before they crossed the boundary from one society to the other. The daily cycles of the solar system are reproduced in the behaviour of all human beings, who need to be asleep for part of it, and awake for the rest of it. For the ill they can have a special significance. The regularity of the cycles of nature, and of the man-made cycles which are intertwined with them, enable people whose future is uncertain to retain some vital certainties. The way in which we reduce uncertainty, and find some order within it, is to make as much as we can of what is predictable. As Marris has said:

> We can impose widely various interpretations on the physical universe, seeing different meanings in it, and still live well enough. What we cannot do is survive without a system of some kind for predicting the course of events.[10]

The turnings of the earth on its axis are the nearest to the predictable that a human being can get. They therefore matter more than ever to people whose future is in so many respects the opposite. When the structure of order is threatened, cling to what is predictable or can be made predictable within it – it could be the golden rule of the sickroom – while always being ready to welcome the surprises, like the letter which unexpectedly has money in it, or the succulent eels a friend has brought in, or a telephone call suggesting an outing, or a daughter who has brought some wallflowers to plant in the garden. And try to accept it when things have to stop. 'When you stop coming, Lesley,' said Kenneth, 'it will be the same. It's another page in the book turned over, a new paragraph, a new beginning.'

Sleep – directly related to the solar system – is a fundamental generator of order. The end of each ordinary day is a time for sleep which is a preparation for another dawn, and each waking up starts off the same familiar sequence as on any other day. Sleep is a little death followed by a little rebirth. The dying people did not stay awake until they died. Even more than other people they needed their sleep each night: they had more to tax them in the day.

> Sometimes if you've had a good night's sleep then you feel good but if you have a fidgety night then you're fidgety all day. (Janet)

Sleep could be difficult to get. In the early period of her illness, Jennifer was so bewildered she could do nothing else but deny that she was ill, and this denied her sleep too. Even though not accepting her illness she feared that if she went to sleep she would not wake up. When she became more realistic, she was able to sleep again, and sleep well. Sleep was also Derek's problem.

> When I wake up at night I get a large blanket and come down to the sitting room. I touch wood, and whistle.

An old lady recommended hot milk with a drop of brandy in it. Whether it was the brandy or the old lady's kindness, it seemed to work.

Harold was exasperated by insomnia because he had always slept so well.

> I've always looked forward to sleep, even in the army when it was difficult enough to get. I could sleep stretched out on a bench on a platform with my army boots wrapped in a towel as a pillow waiting for trains at Shrewsbury. You learnt to sleep standing, crouching. I could sleep through the buzz bombs.

But no longer. He went to bed at 11 p.m. and woke up thinking it was morning to find it was only midnight. After six months of this, his GP gave him some sleeping tablets – 'I don't like to normally but I don't want you to get run down.' It worked well for some months until near the end.

> I had a very bad night last night. It keeps Lilian awake. I had a good night about three nights ago. You have to take the rough with the smooth, I suppose. I wish it were all over – looking forward to the big sleep now.

Waking up and setting the day in motion is the same for almost everyone. In the terraces of East Ham or the tower blocks of Hackney there will be a Harold or a Kenneth, an Alice or a

Jennifer, slowly getting out of bed and having the traditional cup
of tea. If other people look outside to see what the weather is
like, promising a good or bad day in that limited sense, our
people did that as well, and also listened to their insides.

Not so long after looking out of the window comes the first of
the meals which at least bears a resemblance to all the other
breakfasts in a city which is rousing itself from sleep. Then they
move on to the midday and evening meals, meals as regular in
their timing as ever, with the same variations as ever between
them, but without the same appetite. Loss of appetite – something
doctors irritatingly always ask about – is almost more unbearable
for the carers.

Kenneth's wife, Florence, was so used to cooking a hot meal
of chips, greens and meat every evening that she could not accept
things had changed. Being implored by her, Kenneth had to force
it down with as unperturbed a face as he could manage, even
while remembering the stomach pains to come. Jennifer hated to
turn down the food her husband cooked for her – it upset him a
lot when she did – but sometimes she couldn't eat even a mouthful of a dish that he had taken hours to prepare. She just picked
at it.

Alice was still able to cook for herself and it was not always a
humdrum task. She was on her own during the day and was apt
to personalise her food. 'I opened the fridge door,' she said, 'and
looked at this potato and thought "I'll bake you", and I did
and it was lovely.' It was the same with her walking stick. 'I tell
it "I'm sorry, I wish I could do without you". I tell it off. But by
the time I get to the top of the road I want it.'

People ate less and needed smaller portions than before they
got ill. They could eat more if offered less. But the meals could
taste as good as ever, to others as well as oneself. Food was (as
always) a sign of health and a symbol of community with others.
The same Derek who thought that we should use this life on
earth as a testing ground, so that we can make our own way into
eternal life, was happy to test out his skill on a cauliflower cheese
to share with Mrs Litten, the woman he lived with. All his life
he had loved cauliflower cheese.

I buy the cheese sauce in a packet but I also use pieces of
older cheese that have been in the fridge for a period of time
and sincerely believe that this adds to the flavour. I am not in

favour of par-boiling the cauliflower. I like it crisp and crunchy.
The cauliflower should have body to it and I only pray that I
can continue to get it ready. We are having it tonight.

Walter had been living on his own for so many years that he
was thoroughly used to it. Cooking and eating were some of his
main pleasures. 'I was up at 6 a.m. this morning boiling a pig's
head to make brawn. I've one in the freezer as well.' Jack Dickson, the comic from the market family, made a speciality of
bread pudding, offering us a slice when we called – the best bread
pudding we had ever eaten. The interviews became meals.

I know how to look after myself. It's an art. You need to let
the bread get crusty hard, then soak it, then you squeeze every
drop of water out, then mash it with your hands, and then add
spice, margarine and sultanas and sugar.

Cauliflower cheese, brawn and bread pudding were as much (or
more) things to look forward to as they had ever been. Even
with such delights, for most people on their own the day could
drag. 'I'm lucky,' said Dora, 'my daughter comes in at night, at
various times. Tonight it will be 7.30 p.m. It's a long day from
7.45 in the morning. The long day, that's the most difficult thing.'

Routines of medication

By ordinary standards the daily routines also had some unusual
features, related to a common term which they had picked up
from their doctors and which added to the impressiveness of what
was being done for them: the word was 'medication'. The other
word that went with it was not medicines or pills but 'tablets'
which were definitely not tablets of stone. They constituted medication, often elaborate and, with no-one to supervise, they were
in charge of it, and especially about how much and when to take
any tablets that were specifically pain-killers. Being a patient was
a job and this particular job was more theirs than that of their
carers. They also added ordinary tablets or linctuses of their own
that were not on prescription. Arthur Jacobs, the sunny Jewish
widower, was like others in that he had to rouse himself by his
alarm clock at 6 a.m. in order to start punctually on his daily
round of tablets if he was to have a chance of getting into his
mouth before sleep all those prescribed by his doctor. Donald

would not have got through the sixteen large and small tablets
he had to swallow every day if he had not begun at 5.30 a.m.
The six tablets Harold had to start with stuck to the roof of his
mouth and tasted so bitter it was a job to get them down.

The tablets added their own temporal patterning to the day, a
two or three or four hourly sequence of the small, the large, the
round and the oval. It was a matter of pride to have a time-box,
a bit like a diary with containers in it or a clock with each hour
hand pointing to a different lot of tablets. The box converted
space into time and time into medications. Janet explained how
useful this was.

> When I was in the hospice I saw these boxes and I asked if I
> could have one and the Macmillan said it was a good idea.
> They brought me one last Tuesday. It was a great relief. I
> would have my tablets on the side here and if I was talking
> I sometimes didn't know if I'd taken them or not.

Her silent monitor was divided into seven compartments, one
for each day of the week. Each compartment was then sub-
divided for different times of the day and, when they visited, like
the clerks who fill the shelves of supermarkets at night to get
them ready for their consumers, the visiting nurses could parcel
out into these spaces the tablets that had to be taken during the
coming week. All the patient had to do was to check the day
and the time to identify the tablet to take. After a while they did
not even have to look at the box: they could feel their way to
the right compartment, in the dark if necessary. But the final
responsibility was left to those, like Julia, who had at one time
to take her liquid morphine at 5.30 a.m., at the beginning of her
daily steeplechase, then at 9 a.m., at 1 p.m., at 4.30 p.m. and at
9 p.m. People's lives were even more meticulously governed by
the clock than the lives of the hale and the hectic.

For those living on their own, regular visits by neighbours could
serve the same purpose. Walter was alone but a neighbour came
in regularly two or three times a day to bathe his eyes for him,
and for Arthur, also alone, a neighbour arrived every night with
her husband to get him a hot blackcurrant drink – something he
specially liked before going to bed. He appreciated the kindness
and the company even more than the drink. And for almost
everyone the regularity was offset by a precious opportunity
to laugh, even at the conventionally macabre. Harold said,

'Hopefully they'll put me out rather than I become a cabbage. We talk sometimes about it. We have a chat and a laugh about it. I told my daughter-in-law I would come back and haunt her.' There were also the old family jokes to bring up and laugh over again, like the one about the elderly grandmother who says to one of her grandsons:

Will you take me to Arbour Square? I want to get to the police station. I've lost something.

What have you lost, nan?

I've lost my memory and I want to see if they can find it for me.

Weekly cycles

If there was a special regime for the sickroom, for the most part the routines were the general everyday ones, and the same applied to the week. The week is so reassuring partly because (unlike a lifetime) it keeps repeating itself, Monday following Sunday over and over with the splendid precision with which a quartz clock marks the turning over of the minutes. The week was not only marked by the boxes but in scores of other ways as well. Taking it 'day by day' meant day by different day.

The contrasts were sharper than for the healthy, some being ups, and others downs. Small cycles constituted the short-term elements within the longer upward movements which followed on successful treatments, and the longer downward ones as the effect of the treatments wore off. When they were on an up, and feeling better, their morale could bounce upwards; and, even on the days when they were worse, they could, if they were of an optimistic turn of mind, at least look forward to the next mini-recovery. Taking a day at a time was to recognise, along with healthy people, that every day held out at least the possibility of a new dawn. They had not died in the night. They were starting on a new day.

As soon as Kenneth wakes up, he says to himself: 'I hope this is going to be a good day,' and if he hopes it is going to be, or if he is a bit more confident than that and believes it is actually going to be, it will prop him up while he is getting through the coughing fit which he always has when he first gets out of bed in the morning. When it's so bad that his wife looks frightened, he manages to splutter 'all right girl' to her. If he has been coughing too much in bed during the night he will have taken to his chair then and so will 'get up' from there, which still won't mean that he expects a bad day will necessarily follow, one in which he is, say, going to have to take a large quantity of painkillers before the pain 'ebbs away'. If it is going to be a bad day, or a bad patch lasting longer than that, he also remembers that he has bounced back before. So why not again?

If the patient, or the patient and the principal carer, had been completely on their own, never visited and never going out to join in the activities of other people, as if in a kind of solitary or two-person confinement, there could have been more of a tendency for one day to slide imperceptibly into another. But this was not so, even for people who were living quite alone.

Dermot was one of these, on his own in a tiny flat, his nearest relative being his sister in Canada whom we've already mentioned. His Irish parents and uncles and aunts were all dead. When we first saw him, his only visitor was Ellen, a neighbour. She collected his benefit from the Post Office on a Thursday, and did his washing on another day. But after a series of unsuccessful and also painful surgical operations, the Home Care nurse was called in, and from that time on he was joined up to outside society (which he was so soon to leave) in a manner that he had not been for years. Home nurses came twice a week, the Home Care Team doctor once a week; meals-on-wheels came every weekday. The Home Care Team had a telephone installed for him. Even though he did not have friends or relatives to call up, he could now phone for help if it became urgent to get it. The effect was that he gained a weekly timetable from the link that had been made with society. If the day was still the unit of time for him, it had for some purposes been extended into a week by making the days within it at least somewhat different from each other. He did not exactly savour the present but with these differences it was a sight less dreary.

The weekend, for most people, was a future which could be looked forward to with some confidence. It was coming soon, and it had in some ways the same character as it had had during the years of good health. Many of the ill could rejoin society on days when other people were also not working. On Saturday afternoons Donald, for example, kept the radio and the TV on at the same time so that he could turn from one to the other to follow the most exciting bits of the games and horseraces. 'He's a different man on Saturdays,' said Ivy. 'He seems able to rise above the discomfort.' Arthur didn't have that. But he could still look forward to next Saturday. 'Please God, if the weather gets better and I'm still around I shall go out.'

But the weekend was most of all the time when other people could visit, and particularly relatives. On any Saturday or Sunday a high proportion of the cars on British roads must be on such missions.

For Kenneth, Saturday was in its own way as much the high point of his week as for Donald. In Kenneth's family, Saturday lunch was a longstanding family tradition. It wasn't, when we talked to him, as large an affair as it had been. The family had become more dispersed. In the new house there was not so much room. Kenneth could not manage the large numbers who used to come. But three of his four daughters came regularly. Linda had to work on a Saturday so she came every Tuesday night instead, often bringing two king-sized prawns, one of his favourite foods. On the Saturday his other three daughters brought their young children, five between them. Some of his brothers and sisters might drop in too. The same routine was followed every week, and had been since before Kenneth stopped working.

> They all go shopping in the market with the wife and children and then it's the traditional East End pie and mash which they eat there or bring home and eat here. I don't eat much on Saturday, just a snack. There's lots of conversation and maybe reminiscing. Laughter, plenty of that, and occasional tears. They all talk to each other. Problems are aired and solved. Sometimes I fall asleep.

But usually Kenneth maintained his special role as the family's chief problem-solver by staying wide awake. When he was first taken ill, his girls thought they should not come to him with their troubles, as they always had done more than to their mother. He had to tell them and tell them again and again that he wanted them to come to him, on a Saturday, or any other day if they would rather be on their own with him. 'There's nothing wrong with my brain,' he would say. After one session Linda said, 'Thank you, Dad, you've helped a lot.' It was what he wanted to hear.

The Saturday was delightful. But it was also tiring, and Kenneth usually went to bed exhausted, and so did Harold. Sunday was therefore kept as a very quiet day for both of them, with nothing much happening except Sunday dinner.

Plan for attainable goals

One of the greatest setbacks people found was not being able to plan for a longer period ahead than a week or so. Jennifer Barnes, the Afro-Caribbean nurse, said about the time when she was given the news:

> I've lived here 30 years or more and been looking forward to retiring, possibly to Jamaica.

She was being deprived of half of her life that up to then she had been confidently looking forward to. Several of our informants had made similar plans which had to be aborted.

Setbacks or not, they were by no means helpless. When they adopted the second strategy – planning for attainable goals – they could still make a plan but one which took account of their circumstances and set goals which should be attainable. Such plans mattered even more than those they had been forced to give up. They could be invested with a kind of magical significance. If they set themselves a target date it would mean they would survive till then, and after it was reached, could set another which could establish another stepping stone into the future. Fixing their mind, and their resolve, on the target meant there was somewhere for the procession of ordinary days to proceed to. To stay alive until then would itself be an achievement. There was also an element of bargaining in it, as if people were saying to the Fates, let me live till then and you can take me without a struggle.

A birthday was the most obvious occasion to select, especially if it was not too far off. Jack lived alone but he was looking forward to his birthday and his relatives telephoned him about it for months ahead. When it came (his last birthday, as it turned out), his family rallied round wonderfully.

> On my birthday Stella and Kate came around 11.30, then my sister Diane, then two of my daughters and their husbands, then my other nieces from Leyton. In the evening there were about 12 here and around 30 people called in during the day. Ron is my eldest brother. He died. He married Muriel who is

also dead, and they had five children. They were all up here on my birthday, sitting everywhere. I'm the eldest brother now.

Afterwards he thought 'Jane never turned up' with his other sisters; and then he remembered, Jane was dead.

Christmas was even more of a standard target. For all those who had relatives it was a real occasion, to be looked forward to for months and planned for carefully. The patients could not go out to buy presents themselves but they could decide what to buy and commission different relatives to buy them. The day itself was usually a treat, even if sometimes too much so, bringing on a post-Christmas relapse. Kenneth said of a Christmas that he had been determined to last out for:

> The house rang with laughter. There were screams of enjoy-ment from the children. It really rang with happiness and laughter and was absolutely gorgeous. The shining expressions on their faces, the excitement and oh the thrill.

Derek was the only person distressed by Christmas.

> On Monday evening I was in a pub and I got fed up with all the working up to Christmas. There's nothing anymore about the birth of our Lord Jesus Christ.

In addition, people made all kinds of plans which suited just themselves. Jennifer Barnes was not able to retire to Jamaica. She was fated to die in London. But she determined she would go there for a holiday, and also to Virginia, to say a proper goodbye to her mother and other relatives. She would take her son with her. Her husband doubted whether it was wise, fearing she would die on the way. Her doctor was not enthusiastic either.

> In the end I decided I was dying anyway and if I died over there, well that was it. So I went. My mother was pleased to see me. I didn't find it hard on the plane because the wheelchair I was in was carried onto the plane. I spent five days in Jamaica and four weeks in Virginia with my sister.

Most people had set such a target in the last year of their lives, and all but one of them achieved it, whether it was just the sunshine of another summer, a birthday, Christmas, a holiday, a daughter's wedding, the birth of a grandchild. In the hospice when Julia went there another patient was 'trying for her 60th birthday.

She managed it by one day.' One target could be followed by another. Harold, the old soldier, said, 'Last year I just wanted to see Christmas. Then I thought I'd like to see the Trooping of the Colour on June 16. I keep setting sights.' Kenneth said:

> Three things I've got to look forward to. My granddaughter is getting married in July. A great granddaughter or son is being born in August. My youngest daughter is having a baby in September. My objective is to see these things happen.

Which he did.

The exception was Dora Anstey. Her planned holiday was to be in Spain and it was prepared for in the utmost detail, with everything paid for in advance. She was to go with one of her dearest men friends and two others to make up a quartet. They were going to take the tube from Finchley to Waterloo and catch the train from there to Southampton and then a plane to Spain. Discussing the details was almost as much fun as making the journey, perhaps more so because it was not so tiring to her or so worrying to her companions. The holiday was supposed to start on 26 August. Her daughter, with advice from her GP, thought she was not well enough to go. The visit was called off; she died a few days after she should have left. The other two went and returned on 11 September, just in time for the funeral. She had bought new clothes from Marks & Spencer for the holiday. Her daughter returned them to the shop, unworn, and got the money back.

* * *

These people were all struggling to achieve a good enough death. They had all been through the fire. The drugs they took could not stop them being diminished by the disease. They knew they were being killed, slowly. But there was still a good deal to live for, and it was their achievement to have made it so. Dying is strenuous work which demands new skills and new outlooks if independence is to be preserved. All our people were distressed; but they had all, in one degree or another, developed their own philosophies of how to live with a truncated future. They all tried to take each day as it came. It was terrible to be deprived of the future they had thought they would have, but there could be some compensation if the present was more fully savoured as a consequence. In this they have a lesson for those whose bodies have not yet turned against them.

They also knew that how they felt was not only dependent on their bodies but on their spirit. They knew that it was even more fully them – their essence – than their physical sufferings. They also knew that their fighting spirit, and the will to live from which it came, was not in itself captured by the cancer. If it was not totally immune from the disease, it was something separate from their bodies even while that was where it presumably resided. The spirit did not need to weaken as the body weakened but could even get stronger. The spirit was something to hold on to, to be held up by and to be stubbornly proud of. The spirit was relatively timeless – the continuo above which the solemn and the gay were played out. The spirit was not their body; it was what made them more than a body.

Chapter 4

The carer at home

The last chapter was about people's need to feel independent. This did not mean they stood alone. 'There is no such thing as a baby,'[1] said D.W. Winnicott, the psychologist: for every baby there is a mother. Nor is there any such thing as a patient. You are someone's patient. All our people dearly wanted to hang on to as much independence as they could, but for this they needed help from others. They wanted to avoid being helpless. But, being ill, they could not do as much as before. Unless they were alone at home, with far too much independence, they had to combine independence with some dependence on others in a mix that gradually moved towards more dependence.

When they were in a hospital they were the person whom things are done to rather than the person who does. In 1986 22 per cent of all hospital beds were estimated to be taken up by people who would be dead within twelve months, whether due to cancer or other ailments. This suggests that about one-fifth of the cost of the hospital service went on terminal care, a lower proportion than in 1969 when a comparable study was made, mainly because of increased numbers in residential homes and because hospital stays had become shorter.[2]

But even though dying people have not spent quite so long in hospital, they have gone in and out more often. The shorter stays go along with more frequent admissions and more frequent discharges. There has been more switching about between different degrees of independence and dependence, on doctors and nurses in the one setting and relatives in the other, if there are relatives. When dying people are least adaptable they are called on to be more so. No healthy person has to make such sharp adjustments in such short order. The distancing of death from ordinary life means that, unless family members have gone through it before, people have little experience about what to do.

They have to throw over one set of routines and adopt another. Both ways are painful. It was usually a trial to go into hospital. Almost everyone feared they might never come out, even though hospital could be a haven for people without support of the right kind at home. People would say they had been cocky about death at home, and hospital made it more real and more frightening. The ambulance that came to fetch them could seem like a hearse. It was also quite often a trial to come out and have to assume responsibility for yourself once more, without having a doctor or nurse nearby, and also to find how vexing it was to have to do little things like mending the washing machine and dealing with bills and pills on your own. But it was also a release.

> I'm very glad to get away from the hospital with patients dying all the time. I was beginning to feel I couldn't think of anything else. In the normal world, you don't think about death and dying every day, but I began to get absorbed by it.   (Julia)

She had been in the hospice ward of a hospital, and it was a relief to get away from it, even if she was on her own. The responsibility you shirked was also the independence you wanted. You could feel an individual again, instead of a slave under the control, body if not soul, of the benevolent master or mistress whose name was on the board above your bed.

In the hospital you had little more than a toothbrush to call your own. At home it was all yours – the chair you sat in, the bed you were so used to, your clothes, your cup, your own lavatory and your own bath – none of our patients' homes were without piped water. Better than that, you could eat what you liked instead of the hospital food – which was almost universally disliked, partly because it was not their own – and along with that, have a decent fresh cup of tea instead of the substitute tea from a machine which rolls around the wards at times when you don't necessarily want it. It is a mystery why, when in Britain it means so much, the doctor above the bed and the sister beside it do not more often allow patients who are up and about to make tea (and coffee) for themselves and others, at least to supplement the machine.

At home you could be surrounded by objects whose biographies were also your own – objects all the more precious because they had no market value – a German bayonet from the First World War hanging on the wall, sea-shells picked up from a beach in Margate on a vivid holiday in 1933, the picture of a country stream inherited from an aunt, the vase your son won in a fair, a beer mug which was a prize in a darts match, a photograph of West Ham's soccer team in 1957.

At home you could exercise altogether more control. You could shut the front door, and only open it to let in the people you actually wanted to see instead of those who wanted to see you. Medication permitting, you could wake up and get up in accord with the routine you wanted instead of when the nurses wanted; you could have your meals at the times that suited you instead of when the trolley came round; you could rest when you wanted and, commanding silence, go to sleep when you wished; you could telephone who you wanted and know that people would telephone you first if they wanted to come; you could stroke your cats and dogs and play whatever music you wanted; and, if you could muster enough concentration, read a newspaper or book when it suited you. It was no surprise that holidays away from home, when offered by the Home Care Team, were turned down. As Harold said of home, 'I know we can get help straight away.' He might have added, with people we know and who know us.

So at home you could be as much yourself as your illness would allow. Kenneth Chandler said:

> Now every day, every week, every month is a big bonus. Home, that's what it's all about, being here, feeling relaxed, knowing people can come in and feel at ease. That's it, isn't it, knowing you feel comfortable and I can be myself.

At home people could also be more aware of their worries. 'Do you know what I lie thinking about at night?' asked Alice who was a widow, 'I lie there thinking what will happen to my cat if I pass away. My daughter doesn't answer me when I say, "If I go to see Dad what's going to happen to Lulu?".' Alice introduced this roundabout way of talking about her dying because she wanted to say to her daughter that she did not want to go into hospital or die there. When she did try to say it, her daughter changed the subject.

Relatives

What mattered even more was not the space, filled with its memories, but the people sharing it. Whether home was a real haven depended on the relationships within it, and the expectations of those within it about how people should behave – how brave they were, how calm, how querulous, how much they showed their feelings. More than anything else, it depended on the tenderness within it.

Eight of the patients had a relative living with them – five a spouse, one, although unmarried, a partner, one a mother and one a daughter. Four were living on their own but with daughters or sons very much on the scene. Two were living quite alone. It was, as usual for carers, very notable that where there was a principal carer, all but two of them (Barnes and Bliss) were women. In the sickroom gender-typing of roles is still very marked. In families, caring 'flows out of the customary responsibilities',[3] as do the excuses for not taking responsibility. Full-time employment was an excuse, or a reason, for not taking much of a part as a carer, and so was living some distance away.[4]

Friends mostly drifted away, paying visits at the start of the illness and tailing off thereafter. Friends from work no longer had that bond in common. Friends from the pub or club no longer were the same. There could be less and less to talk about; people who had been seen quite frequently became 'telephone friends', ringing to enquire now and then how things were. On the whole the main work was left to the family who had so much more of the past to share. The family also had a common interest in the present. However sadly, they were together following the course of the disease week by week.

The carers could not avoid a series of adjustments in their own lives and ideas which were almost as far-reaching for them as for their patients. If it is so wearing for the dying person to get his mind round the fact that soon he will not exist (or, if at all, in a very different form), it can be even more so for the carers to imagine a world from which the dying person, who is so real to them, has vanished, leaving them to face a life without him or her. If they had come to take it for granted that the patient would always be there to look after them, how could they accept the reversal? If they could not, denial of the truth was as much (perhaps even more) their first defence as it was for the patient.

Some spouses said they communicated by telepathy. They did not have to talk. But how to imagine a future without any message waiting for them from the other end of the telepathy?

The strain was all the greater on both sides because the patient could change almost as rapidly as a new-born infant at the other end of the age spectrum. The patient was liable to become a different person, especially in the first phases of the illness while still suffering from shock, not only changing physically but also in behaviour, becoming withdrawn, grumpy, demanding, when they had not been like that when well. If this had happened in ordinary times, it could have been openly discussed. But now that the changelings have to be treated with special consideration, the carers' queries and resentments have to be bottled up.

So there had to be adjustment all round by patients and carers. Each family had only its own experience to call upon, its own ways of dealing, or not dealing, with crises. Trying to cope with the new and supreme one, they were liable to react to the new crisis as they had to others and follow their old family patterns.

> There may be rules within the awareness of the family which come to be openly stated. 'We are a democratic family in which everyone has a right to be heard.' 'We all share the work, and everyone knows what jobs they have to do.' 'We don't believe in rules and want everyone to do as they like.' There are also rules which are not stated: 'Mother does all the nasty jobs'; 'No one has to take any notice of father'; 'We never show how angry we are with each other'. Sometimes these spoken and unspoken rules appear to be in conflict with each other. There are also other rules which operate outside the conscious awareness of the family altogether.[5]

In the same vein Hinton has shown that 'there is support for the frequent impression that a patient's previous manner of living influences the way he dies', in particular 'the capacity of facing or not facing problems in the past affected the mood during the terminal illness',[6] with those who had been unable to cope being the same when they most needed not to be, and those who had been able continuing to be able. Jack Dickson coped when he lost his wife soon after the birth of his daughters and when, later on, he lost his market stall after being knocked down by a lorry. He was matter of fact about it; he did not complain. On the other hand, Marjorie wondered about the cancer she had been told she had – 'is there anything there?' – and behaved as though there wasn't, as she had always dealt with setbacks. Carol ignored her first symptoms as she had ignored other painful circumstances. Kenneth's calm may have been learnt from his earlier adversities.

Traditional families

It was easiest to continue as in the past in the kind of family which we think of as traditional East London, in one or other of its types. We do not say the traditional East London family because in that, according to some previous books from the Institute of Community Studies,[7] the mother was the dominant figure rather than the father, whereas in both the families we are going to cite now – the Chandlers and the Allens – the man, at least when he was at home for a long stretch, was dominant and remained so throughout his illness. Even while he was dying, he was the household's undisputed head. Perhaps partly because he was dying, his word was more law than ever. The Knights were very similar, as we described them before.

This must have been so over the whole of the fifty years or so of their marriages. The husbands had brought in most of the money even when it was supplemented by their wives, and their wives had looked after their husbands and children when they were ill, which was very frequently for Kenneth and not infrequently for Harold. Terrible as it was for Lilian and Florence when their husbands became ill with cancer, at least they did not have to change their role of carer, housekeeper, cook, companion. They did not know in advance how to do the more demanding nursing they now had to do – this had to be learned the hard way, by doing it and failing and taking advice and doing it again; but they did know how to look after a home and make a dying husband not only comfortable but feel as much respected, as loved, as he had ever been. If anyone in East London could choose the setting in which to endure a long-drawn-out illness without too much misery, and with some compensation for the inevitable setback, he would be a man and at home. For a good enough death he would be hard put to do better than Harold Allen or Kenneth Chandler or their like.

A further advantage was their close-knit extended families, or as close-knit as they could be, given their geographical scatter. At the time of the previous studies in the early 1950s, the

extended families would not just have existed, they would also
have been local. This would have been still better for both husband and wife. But despite changes over the last four decades,
the wives in our study were strongly supported as mothers, sisters
and sisters-in-law. The Allens had three grown-up children and
eight grandchildren. Lilian also had two sisters, one still alive,
while Harold had a half-brother and a half-sister. The children
and grandchildren visited often and could be called up for any
service. In this respect the Chandlers were even better off. They
had four daughters for Kenneth to be proud of (the pride being
more than reciprocated) and six noisy but much-loved grandchildren. The family broke the common rule that affection
descends more readily than it ascends. When his whole extended
family came together from their furthest outreaches, as they did
at his funeral, nearly a hundred of them turned up in black
dresses and black suits. The extended family was as much a
support for Florence as it was for Lilian, as well as for their
husbands. They were surrounded with well-wishers, many of
whom they had known for a good part of their lives – too
much so for Florence at around the time of Kenneth's death. His
relatives insisted on turning up when she least wanted them.

The Allens

Without the extended family, Harold might have died a year
before he did. The doctors expected him to. Lilian expected him
to. The children and siblings expected him to, and had been to
say their goodbyes in the hospital. The turnabout seemed like a
miracle. Lilian was an active agent of it, ready to take up again
the burdens of caring for Harold at home partly because she
knew she would not have to carry them on her own.

During what were thought to be his last days he had a distressing experience which proved a blessing, though, at first, very
much in disguise. Harold had nothing but praise for the day
nurses and the opposite for the agency nurses on night duty – as
we also heard from other people. The night nurses would put his
medication on the table by his bed and expect him to take it
himself although he was too weak to reach it. He would say,
'Please pull me up because I can't take my medication like this.'
One nurse came along, saw he hadn't taken his pills, opened his
mouth and threw them down his throat. From then on, he went

on pill-strike. He refused all medication and determined he would
die. But before that he said to Lilian, rather casually, that he was
sorry he would not be able to die at home. He couldn't get out
of his bed and walk (as Alice had done). But Lilian wondered
whether he was right and went immediately to see his GP, Dr
Clayton. Could Harold come home? she asked. In hospital he
was as sad as he could be.

The admirable doctor, without committing himself, said 'all
things are possible' and went off right away to the hospital. The
ward sister was exceedingly unhelpful. A mere GP has no standing in a hospital; he's standing on someone else's turf. She did
not want to let Harold go – he had in a sense become the
hospital's property – even though there was nothing they could
do for him, nor indeed for many other people who were dying.
The common practice of isolating them to die on their own in
side-wards can be the worst thing to do. Dr Clayton, when asked
about it later, remembered during his training a patient who was
dying and did not know it. He asked the consultant, 'Shall I tell
him?' The consultant replied in an off-hand way, 'No, don't
bother.' It had been very educative: Dr Clayton was unusual in
taking it as an object lesson in what *not* to do.

But he persuaded the hospital authorities to let his patient go
by explaining that he himself would call on Harold twice a day;
the Home Care Team would be brought in and the district nurse.
The sister's most worrying question was whether Harold would
survive until he settled back home. Everyone did their best to
ensure he would. The family, in Lilian's words, 'rallied round'.
Lilian's sister, the person she could most easily talk to because
her own husband had died of cancer a few years before, had
been staying with her for what could have been the last week of
Harold's life. When it wasn't, and Harold was coming home, she
stayed on. Lilian's daughter from Exeter, a nurse herself, also
came to stay for two weeks.

Dr Clayton, the hero, brought off an organisational tour de
force. His practice nurse procured a hospital bed and a hoist to
go in the ground-floor sitting room, a supple mattress and a
sheepskin to prevent bed-sores. He alerted the Home Care
service. An auxiliary nurse called to give Harold a blanket bath.
District nurses came twice a day to lift him out of bed in the
morning and lift him back in the evening – something that to
begin with Lilian could not do on her own. Dr Clayton arrived

once or twice a day and, in case there was an emergency, gave
Lilian his home and bleeper numbers as well as his surgery
number. It was not surprising that, with all this marvellous fuss,
the pill-throwing night nurse was soon almost forgotten. Harold
began to recover his strength. He determined to last out over
Christmas. He succeeded in that; he was still alive the following Christmas.

Dr Clayton told Harold what had happened. The cancer in the
pancreas had proved inoperable. He had not been told this in
the hospital. Harold laughed because for ten years he had been
struggling with a heart and lung condition. Perhaps he was going
to die of something else! Thus began a series of conversations
with the GP in which they were completely open with each other,
and most of what Harold heard he passed on to his family.

He talked about his coming death to his grandchildren and
made them laugh by saying he would come back to haunt them.
In the same vein Lilian told him that one day she'd come into
the room and only his pyjamas would be there, walking around
without him inside them. He himself would have faded away – a
reference to a saying he was fond of – 'old soldiers never die,
they only fade away'. Harold said he'd seen so much death in
the war that he couldn't be afraid of it. He'd had a charmed life
and he thought it was continuing. He'd been indestructible. In a
troopship in a great storm 180 miles out in the Atlantic, they had
been bombed. The ship was hit on two quarters, sprang a leak
and caught fire. A train was bombed just after he got off it. A
hotel was bombed but his bedroom was spared. He was in the
frontline in Normandy when it was attacked by a plane dropping
strike bombs. The enemy plane swooped down the line but strad-
dled him, one bomb dropping 20 yards behind and another a few
yards in front. 'I was saved for something else' – for Dr Clayton
and Lilian to save him again from the death he had escaped
before.

In his last year of life he saw a good deal of his children and
grandchildren. There was a particular link with one grandson.
Before the war Harold had been trained as a french polisher and
he was prouder of that trade than of the Inland Revenue,
where he had worked as a clerk from the time he was demobil-
ised. He kept his hand in by doing a professional job on the pews
in his church. So he was happy when this grandson took up the

same occupation, skipping a generation but continuing a family tradition.

That was very agreeable; less so was having to sit in a chair and watch his sons and son-in-law fixing the doors and windows which he would like to have done himself. He was happy for Lilian to do the cooking, though he sometimes minded her being away from him in the kitchen. But he knew that, when she was there, she had the radio on so low that she would hear his stick banging on the floor next door if he wanted her. Cooking had always been her job. But he did mind not being able to help with the 'man's work', though also pleased that he had sons and a son-in-law who would do what he could now only plan for

Once, when one of us called to see Harold, the house was like a builder's yard, with Harold sitting in the middle of it. He rented the house from his son-in-law in Exeter who, as the owner, had a special interest in improving the property. He wanted to do it after Harold died, but Harold insisted it be done before. On that day he was there installing new modern windows and window frames throughout. The old windows could not be opened by Lilian but could be by a determined burglar. They did not keep the noise out or the heat in. This quadruple disadvantage was now being remedied by having double-glazed windows and french doors which could be opened and also locked. Harold's son from Croydon, a railwayman, came to clean up. Another son who lived at Billericay installed the double-glazing, and intended to do the same with a new front door which would have three locks and an alarm. 'The wife will be safe when I go – fortified.' She wouldn't ever have to move, although Harold had told her minutely that it would be a good idea, after staying at home for two or three weeks after the funeral, to go down to Exeter for a month to 'break it up'. Sitting in his special armchair Harold was, genially, considerately, humorously, still being treated, and considering himself, as the head of the household, in life and beyond.

The Chandlers

The Chandlers were similar. The cancer had not made so much difference to them since it followed a whole string of disasters, going back to the Second World War. Kenneth had been badly wounded in the landings in Europe and, after months of painful operations, when his leg was amputated that had been the first great trial for his wife, Florence. She had to accept that Kenneth would have trouble with his health and would need looking after. He did and she did. His tin leg became part of the education, first of his children – they had four daughters – and then of his six grandchildren from 21 down to 2. When each generation of children was young:

> I tell them I've got little men working in my leg and their eyes open wide with wonder. I tell them you can't see them but you can touch them. They put their fingers in the hole on one side and I put my hand in on the other. They often come up and say 'feel the little men grandad?'

After that came the trouble with his lungs – brought on, the doctors said, by the strain of losing his leg. He had open heart surgery, but his breathing remained so bad that it was his chief problem, even more than his cancer. 'It's there 24 hours a day and I can't get away from it. The cancer I can put at the back of my mind although I know one day it'll catch up with me.'

Florence had learned to cope with Kenneth's disabilities and also to fall in with Kenneth's role of hero. This had kept him going through adversities which, taken singly, would have been enough to kill almost anyone. To his whole family he was a hero and he had been made even more so by his cancer – if there were a Victoria Cross for bravery in illness his family would have had no hesitation in awarding it to Kenneth. This helped him and his wife to bear their numerous setbacks. He made light of them, although when the dreaded word, cancer, was first uttered in the house it caused great misgiving. He was able to appear so brave, he explained to us, partly because, without telling Florence, he regularly unburdened himself late at night to his dead mother and brother and sought a blessing from them.

That apart, Kenneth and his family were open enough with each other. Their GP was also helpful and Kenneth's daughters as well as Florence knew the doctors at the nearby London Hospital almost as well as he did himself. Scattered all over greater East London and out into Essex, they could not come in every day to see their parents in the Isle of Dogs, but they phoned regularly and drove up when there was any trouble. Kenneth's own brothers and sisters – eleven of them – had mostly lived near Reading. The war was responsible. The family had

been evacuated from the Isle of Dogs to near Reading at the
first threat of bombing. Kenneth's beloved mother had stayed on
and many of his brothers and sisters. The Queen's Arms on the
Bath Road was the meeting place for the whole extended family
whenever a daughter or son got married. Kenneth went to stay
there with one of his sisters, and they were as solicitous as
Florence. Once when bleeding started up

> I wanted to burn my underwear but she insisted on washing
> them. She said it was no problem, she'd had all this with Ron.
> I said, 'Please don't fuss', but she dithered around me.

Even his mother's death had not broken up the network. Kenneth's cancer acted rather like birthdays in other families – it
brought people together. This was because Kenneth had taken
the place of his mother at the centre of the family. He loved
people to come to him for advice and his sympathy brought
people to him, including his remaining brothers and sisters. Or
they just got together and recalled old times.

> On Sunday my brother, Gerald, and his wife and his eldest
> son and wife and two children came and my younger brother
> Maurice and his two daughters and one of my younger sisters,
> Marjorie. All domestic you know and then slowly we drifted
> back and reminisced. A lot of them don't remember quite up
> to the war.

Florence was so engrossed in her husband's illness that she had
less time for her own siblings and other relatives, even for her
sister who died before Kenneth and without Florence being able
to do for her all she would have liked – indeed far from it.

The Barnes family

Another of our patients was part of an extended family but
with a much wider geographical reach than the Allens and the
Chandlers, with tentacles stretching to Jamaica and Virginia. The
chief difference, though, was not the extended family but the sex
of the patient. Jennifer had the cancer, not John.

To begin with, she said, John would not talk at all, partly
because she herself was rather tongue-tied as well. He was withdrawn because he felt helpless and guilty because he could not
do more. John had always been a loner. She could visualise him,

unhappily, unhappy after she had died. 'He'll sit here and not answer the door, I know him.' She was right as far as we were concerned. He did not respond to our phone calls after she died. Early on, Jennifer had told her sister-in-law that she would have to come over and take John bodily away with her to look after him.

Gradually, once Jennifer had got over the shock of it (as we described in Chapter 3), she began to encourage her husband to talk a little more openly. He joined in when friends came to find out how she was and did not dry up completely on the subject of her cancer when they had gone. 'So what was taboo at one time isn't taboo any more.'

Their greater openness with each other made it easier to accomplish the reversal of roles. To begin with, the Barnes had continued rather as they had done before. Jennifer did not give up work right away, nor did her husband. But if he was to do more in the home it would be that much more difficult if he continued to work, especially when she herself could no longer do so. Fortunately for the family, John's employer, a local authority, was very considerate. He was near retirement and, on the production of a doctor's letter explaining why he was now needed at home, he was allowed to take indefinite sick leave, and then a pension.

Released from his old job, John did not hold back from his new one – not enough, as it happened – but threw himself into it with a will. He had always enjoyed cooking – in that respect it was easier for him than it would have been for many men. But he bought too much and cooked too much. Like Florence and Lilian, he could not believe his partner now had no appetite. Jennifer tried not to disappoint him by eating as much as she could, just as Kenneth did in order not to hurt Florence's feelings. But (as we said) there were limits.

> It used to hurt him when I turned it away because he was trying his best, not that I didn't appreciate it but I didn't have the appetite.

He did not want her to do anything except just sit, as though she, who had once been the centre of the family, always on the go, the manager, was now a fragile doll who could not do anything lest she break into pieces. Her problem was not to accelerate the reversal of roles but to put a brake on it – persuade him that she could still do some of the things she had always done. She wanted to feel she was still of some use, not a doll. After many weeks she won him round. When she announced that 'last Sunday he allowed me to cook dinner' she was as delighted as if she had been promoted at work.

She promised John to stop if she got tired. But she now felt less tired rather than more. 'The space I needed, I'm getting it now. With our understanding of each other, the space has come without really knowing it.' In other ways, too, she did not need to act more as the sick person than she felt. She went out to shop, to visit friends and to church.

> I used to lie on top of the bedclothes. John would tuck me in. He had to do everything. He doesn't have to now. I'm happier and it makes him happier.

It was even more remarkable to have come to terms after a struggle with the new division of labour than to go on, as the Allens did, as they had done before the illness.

Jennifer's son, Lee, was more of a problem. He could not cope and she could not tell him how to. He kept away, was very cold, withdrawn, would not look at her. He wouldn't talk to her or anyone else about the illness. She remembered what she had done when her five-day-old baby daughter had died. She hadn't wanted Lee to be afraid of death as some children are when their parents hush it up. So she brought baby clothes – a frock and a bonnet – to the mortuary, dressed the baby in them and showed Lee his dead sister, explaining who she was. Lee has remembered it vividly and, apparently, not as a frightening experience. Even so she was afraid it could be that memory. Or it could be her illness had revived the sadness of two years before when a child-minder he called his nan had died. He had been very fond of her. She had looked after him as a child in the afternoons after school since he was 5. He had seen her in great pain and, most likely, thought that would be the same again, with his mother.

> What's coming ahead I can't see, so I can't advise him. He's got to come to terms with things himself. I don't understand it myself so I can't explain it to him. I'm learning each day to cope with each day and he'll have to do the same thing.

There was so much to 'explain', or try to, besides the answer or the non-answer to the clock-question about how long she had

got. Why me? Why to this family? What can happen to relationships that one thought would last and last? What and where are
the feelings that the occasion calls for? How to stop them being
overwhelming? Why should I feel guilty? And what is the meaning of it all? The questions did not go away – all the more
because there were no answers. But slowly she managed to draw
out John but not Lee. Carol's daughter, also a teenager, remained
rather aloof throughout.

Jennifer could not stop herself worrying whether John would be
able to manage when she had gone, although she was reassured a
little by seeing him cook and look after the house. She had always
been the organiser.

> He's going to be left behind. I suppose he'll learn and friends
> will help but he's going to be on his own. I can't help him
> that way. He's a person who will withdraw from society – that
> worries me.

In the same way, Walter worried whether his son would be able
to cook and Harold for Lilian's safety when he was no longer
there.

The Rahmans

Another of our patients – Janet Rahman – was like Jennifer in
living with her husband, but in unusual circumstances because
she was not only with him but also with his second 'wife', as she
was regarded in Muslim custom. There was therefore no necessity
for Mr Rahman to do as Mr Barnes did and become a house-
husband and carer. His second wife had a job in a surveyor's firm
but when she was at home she could look after his first wife,
aided by Janet's daughter. If she had been well, the two wives
might have managed to get on, as happens in Muslim households,
even though Janet herself was brought up in England and was
not a Muslim. But with the illness it was difficult on both sides,
and especially for Janet. There was no longer any obvious place
for Janet in the family or in the household, except in her own
room; and it was there she stayed for most of the time, very
much alone and sometimes panicky. One tension in the family,
to add to the others, stemmed from religion, the Muslim attitude to death being much more stoical.

No full-time carers

The stock notion of a family is still that it contains a man and a woman and children, even though the children may have left home. Thought of in that way, the four people we have mentioned so far in this chapter were the only ones in such a family. All the others were without wives or husbands or other carers who could devote all their time to the new vocation. They had little left of their family of origin or never formed such a family as adults or, if they had, it had left little or no trace on how they were living when we saw them.

Two were in mother–daughter households, with the daughter (Carol Taylor) being the patient in one of them and the mother (Dora Anstey) the patient in the other. Neither Carol nor Dora had husbands living with them. Carol was separated; Dora was a widow. Their problems largely stemmed from their having only part-time carers. We described Carol's situation in Chapter 2. Her mother was amazing. She did as much as she could for her daughter. But she gave up one of her three part-time jobs, persevering with the other two in order to bring in enough money for the household. At the age of 76 she managed to combine both her paid job and her unpaid – and this after she had been stricken by a string of family deaths. She had been more attached to another of her daughters than to Carol, and Carol knew that.

Dora Anstey was the other way around, a mother looked after by her daughters, especially by one of them, Jackie. They had not been close to their mother, partly because Dora had been secretive about her relationships with other men. She would not say who the father of the third sister was, refusing even to show her birth certificate. Both daughters were unable to feel the love their mother was asking of them and guilty because they could not.

Jackie, estranged from her husband, came to live with her mother and looked after her early morning and evening. As Dora became more dependent, another daughter, Debbie, joined in, but she didn't live with them until the very last weeks. Both in full-time work, their caring role put an extra strain on them. They boxed and coxed with each other and with their work, one staying at home while the other went to the office. Their mother's battle with death upset, distressed and exhausted them emotionally, and threatened to undermine the two sisters' own close relationship with each other. As for the third sister, she would have little to do with them or her mother, alive or dead. Her uncertain parenthood remained the barrier it had always been.

Most of the other people had a child or children, like Dora, but children who were not living with them. They were widowers and widows unable to form joint households with their children, either by living with them or by the children coming back home. They were alike in grieving for the husbands and wives who had died and also in having children who could give them some support.

Alice Colyer's daughter did least, not only because she had a full-time job, but her mother was so easy-going and contented. But as she lived only a few minutes' away, she came in regularly to bring the shopping she did twice a week at Marks & Spencer. There were always enough ready-cooked dishes for all her mother's meals. Eddie Bliss did much more for his 93-year-old father. He lived nearby and he was in and out of his father's flat almost daily. When one of us called for an interview Eddie was hoovering the hall after having just finished washing the kitchen floor. Jack Dickson's surviving daughters visited him every weekend to shop and clean and rang him several times during the week. Even so, the widows and widowers on their own were all lonely, at times very. They were dying second when they would have had it easier if they'd died first, before their spouses. But at least they did not have to go through readjustments in very close, lifetime relationships like those who were married.

Arthur Jacobs was unusual, and not just in having been widowed twice. He had been living quietly on his own, a recluse, lonely after the death of his second wife, estranged from the sons he had had with his first wife and from his step-daughters by his second. But his cancer brought his family together again, and not in order to get a share in his property, for, as far as we know, he had none. Being so near to death, he was forgiven. His step-daughter who lived across the street started to call in every day. A son did so almost as often. Another son appeared from Chester. Arthur's own children and his step-children met for the first time. He thought of phoning another son in Australia to say goodbye, even though there had been an almost complete rift. In his little flat, from having no family he suddenly had almost too much of one.

The principle of substitution works in many families. If a spouse is available as a full-time carer, other members of the family

matter if only in a supporting role. But if the person who would
have been a full-time carer is no more, or never existed, children
and other relatives move up to do more. It is the reverse of what
can happen when parents as the principal carers for children are
incapacitated or absent: a grandparent may step in as a substitute.
If there is no grandparent it can be an uncle or aunt, abiding by
more or less the same priorities of the moral economy as in the
rules which determine who shall be the next-of-kin and inherit
an estate in the event of intestacy. At the other end of life when
the spouse is absent it is not the still older people who step in –
although that happened with Carol – but the younger.

Neighbours

Did neighbours help? Did the same principle of substitution apply
to them? Were they not in evidence whenever there were relatives? And did they appear where there were no relatives, or
none nearby?

The Allens were (as we have seen) a close-knit family and
neighbours were barely mentioned. They spoke of them as having
had them once. Neighbours would have helped 'in the old days'
(before the great outgoing from East London and the great
incoming of others from Bangladesh, the West Indies, India and
Africa), when people grew up together and lived together for
long periods in the same street or locality, and they would have
done so even if husband and wife had both been alive. Lilian
would have agreed with Ivy Knight.

> The old camaraderie of the street is lost now because of immi-
> gration. The Indian women don't speak English. They've a lot
> to share with us but can't. They don't want to be integrated,
> they make no effort. The community has gone; I do miss that.
> When I was young, the streets were like small villages, like a
> big family you could turn to. A lot of people feel like I do
> and some feel very bitter about it. They (Indians) cling
> together and can't drop their old ways. I do miss all that,
> especially now that women don't like going out after dark. It
> makes the evening very long.

The Allens thought the help would not be on offer – or not to
the extent it once would have been – even if they had wanted it.
The Chandlers thought that neighbours would have been helpful

enough if there had been the opportunity and the need. Their immediate neighbours had said to bang on the wall if they needed anything. 'Just tell us. You know where we are' – that is, sitting watching the same television programme on the other side of the party wall. But Kenneth did not want them calling in for tea and a chat. He feared they would tire him; he wanted to reserve his energies for his children and grandchildren. Both he and Florence were sure that if they did have a need they would call (literally, on the indispensable telephone) on their more distant daughters rather than on next door. Thus summoned, a daughter would speed through the streets and be there within the hour.

Dora was the only one with a live-in carer – a daughter as we've seen – who had help from her neighbours. Dora's were of long standing, having moved into the block with her forty years before. They knew Dora was on her own in the daytime.

> My neighbour calls by most mornings and buys things for me and comes in and sits with me. We moved into these flats together. I used to know a lot of people here. When the children are very young, you get to know people but as they are older you lose touch. I used to work and people moved away. Now I know them to say hello but I don't know them intimately.
>
> I might sit outside and talk to the neighbours during the day. I've got an old friend upstairs. I can talk to her. I see her most days for five minutes or so. I've been lucky these last couple of weeks because she's had decorators around and so she's spent a lot of time down here. I've been spoiled.

When Dora came out of hospital after intensive chemotherapy, she was too ill to be on her own. Her neighbours could only do so much.

> When I was frightened, she [her daughter] engaged a young woman to come every morning to stay and talk with me. Different people from round about here would come in the afternoons to be with me.

Whatever social contact Dora had, it wasn't enough.

> What I would like is someone to come and sit with me and talk.

Neighbours to the fore

It was different again for people living on their own, such as
Jack, Arthur and Walter. They were not without some support
from relatives. But they needed more than that and they did, in
fact, all get help from women neighbours who were more sup-
plements than substitutes for family. Jack's helpmate lived on the
floor above, paid the rent for him every Thursday and collected
his pension. She was acting in accord with the normal obligations
in the sort of community life he had been brought up in.

> My neighbour drops in to collect my pension, do washing. She
> calls in any time to see if I'm wanting anything, like a paper
> from the shop. Neighbourly, like one should be.
>   She lived in my turning in the market. I've known her since
> the war. My family knew her too. She's about 65. She generally
> calls in every evening as well, around 8.30–8.45, to see if I
> need anything. She doesn't do it at the weekend but she comes
> down on Saturday and has a chat with my daughters. She
> drops in when she knows they'll be here and has a few words.

So Jack's daughters had someone they'd known since their childhood to keep an eye on him.

Arthur and Walter saw their neighbours as more than that. For
Arthur, Myra was his 'angel'; for Walter, his neighbour, Mavis,
was his 'bubba'. Arthur's angel had kept a watchful eye out for
him long before his family was re-united. He'd known Myra
for the seven years he'd been living in his flat and wouldn't have
a word said against her. She was married but her family had
grown up and moved away.

> My neighbour takes the prescription to the chemist for me.
> Outside it's a communal yard and we all sit there in the
> summer. She pops in three times a day, morning, lunch and
> night, and in the evening she comes with her husband and a
> drink of blackcurrant. I don't like her to do it because she
> won't take a halfpenny off me. I feel terrible over it. She
> bought some cheese that I like, she made a special trip to a
> shop for me. Tonight she'll come in with her husband for
> a chat. That's my angel. Myra is chatty. She knows people and
> likes to help people. She's a happy enough soul.

Walter's 'bubba' was a local lady from the same landing; she could open her door and be into his flat in a flash. Walter's door was usually open, on the catch or ajar, if the weather was warm. She once popped in while we were there just to see if there was anything Walter wanted.

> A lovely woman. She'll bring me a pot of jam, anything. She pops in and out as if she's me sister. When she's going shopping she asks if I want anything brought back, every day, yes every day. I call her my 'bubba'. She comes in two or three times a day to dress my eyes. She's like a confessional. Her husband's been here as long as I have. He died. He was a very nice man. I don't make a fuss, I accept it. I'm not young any more.

Walter also had a friend, Fred, also on the same landing who called in regularly, the only man mentioned. Fred once stayed for a chat when we were there. He was Walter's scribe.

> Fred does all my pension books and letters, etc. and writes them all out for me. He's very good.

Alice, Jack, Arthur and Walter Bliss had relatives who called in at regular intervals. Another three people living on their own when they first got cancer had no children and very little or no contact with any relatives still alive. Dermot was one of them. He had no family in England. His neighbour, Ellen, lived alone on the landing above and he must have known her for about eight years.

> I met Ellen after I moved in. She's Irish. She goes to church every morning. She's a very Christian woman. She's about 80. Every year for the last eight years she's brought in Christmas dinner for me.

Ellen did Dermot's washing; he declined a home help because of her assistance. She came in a couple of times a week and got him 'a bit of stuff – she keeps bringing me in food'. She also looked after the bed-ridden lady who lived next door to Dermot and brought her a paper every day. She visited him regularly, several times a week during his last stay in hospital and in his last days in the hospice. One of us met her briefly in the London Hospital, a slow heavy-looking woman, large against Dermot's small frame, and shy. The same day she went off to the Post Office to get his pension.

Derek Wood was divorced from his wife and cut off from their children. But he found a neighbour who became much more than a neighbour, a wife, or as good as one, when he was taken ill.

He had been on his own for most of his recent life and had been scared, when he got cancer, that he would fall down the stairs and there would be no-one with him to find him or help him if he was still alive. It was partly because he was in such dire straits that a woman whom he already knew a little invited him to move in. He at once became less anxious. It was a joy to be living with someone again and someone who cherished him as much as he did her. The cancer had in a way done them a good turn in bringing them together in the same house – it was one of the happiest homes we visited. The only trouble was the criticism they had to face from friends and family for 'living in sin'. This would have been resolved if they had been able to do as they intended and marry at Easter. He died a short time before the wedding.

As for our last patient, Julia, her friend Maria used to work in the same hospital. Later, she bought a flat near Julia's and they grew closer and closer, like sisters, or more so.

> I haven't done all that much. Julia looked after herself mostly. It's only in the last year that that has become impossible or more difficult. I started by just doing the heavy shopping for her and I've gradually done more.

Maria accompanied Julia to shop in the West End, talked over her religious experience with her, went with her to the local church where Julia threw Holy Water over herself, took days off work and struggled across London to visit the far-off orthopaedic hospital, bought food when the home help hadn't. Later in Julia's illness she always came over with a cooked meal which they ate together in the evening; she emptied ashtrays as a reflex action whenever she walked into Julia's flat and, for a while, co-ordinated the many visitors who called on Julia at hospital. Other friends helped too, in particular Daphne, buying clothes and nightdresses to fit Julia's expanding frame, visiting her regularly, accompanying her to outpatients. Both women had to take time off work to do this, even time off for their own illness as the strain began to take its toll on them. Maria was exceptional, but like some other neighbours, in becoming an eager substitute for the family and on the model of the family. In the final stages of illness when her family appeared by the bedside, neighbours like Myra and Ellen deferred to them and were less often seen around.

Access to support services

Whether or not they had caring relatives or neighbours, all our people had support from the Home Care service. The Knights were not alone in feeling that: 'Directly the Macmillan came on the scene there was a calm for both of us.' There was the additional comfort that the nurses seemed to know what everyone needed. Ivy Knight, again, said, 'If you mention anything, they always seem to have something to hand to help. It's this whole feeling of care and concern. It's everything.'

A call from the Home Care Team to the social service department, or anywhere, could do more than an individual, even an individual who was dying. The nurses knew where to go for everything – for a loan of wheelchairs, hoists, ripple mattresses, walking frames; who to get on to for adaptations like rails for the bath and stair lifts which can make home more manageable; where to go for home helps or subsidised telephones or taxi cards or sound alarms. Dying is a new way of life; without help, people can hardly make a decent go of it.[8]

A hospital could play the same part. In this respect the Royal Marsden Hospital, a special hospital for cancer patients, seemed to be particularly prized. For Jack Dickson 'Even the cleaners were like ladies.' He found when he got back home that the Marsden had laid on the Home Care Team for him; a phone he'd not been able to afford for himself; a bed rest; a rail on the bath. If such miracles were possible, perhaps he'd even find himself day-by-day getting stronger.

People could also get advice from the Home Care Team about money, tight for almost everyone. Once the sickness benefit of the younger people ran out, they could (if they were insured) get invalidity benefit which could be topped up by Income Support. But they needed help in filling up the forms. The older people at least had pensions which did not go down because they were dying. In one respect, the support improved while our enquiry was in progress. Patients could get an Attendance Allowance more or less immediately on applying for it. There is a higher rate for patients who need to be looked after at night as well as by day. But fear of bureaucracy was a deterrent. 'I never applied for that,' said Lilian Allen. 'It takes time to go through and if they've died before it's gone through they don't give it backdated.'

Some patients were worried about money, for instance about the housing benefit they were entitled to if they were council tenants and their incomes were low. Jack Dickson was driven to distraction by having a much higher rent suddenly demanded by the housing department without being able to get any adjustment from the Department of Social Security. He could no longer go round to the local housing office to 'sort it out' or 'sort them out', and the government office which had once been local had now moved to Scotland. Its new, rationalised and computerised system spewed out to Jack only quite unintelligible and exasperating notices. Why did his few pounds of housing benefit in Spitalfields have to be negotiated in Scotland?

Where to die?

All in all, our people were fortunate to have Home Care nurses and social workers to help them find their way around the welfare state as well as in many other ways. But home care or no home care, at the end of their illness they still sometimes faced one last crucial choice. Where to die?

Very many people (according to various surveys) would rather not just stay at home over the long haul but die at home too. In one recent study the initial preference of 58 per cent of people for their place of death was home, with hospital and hospice tying at a low level for the rest.[9] Only half of those who expressed a preference for home eventually died there. Another study of patients who died in a hospital or hospice found that only 24 per cent of those in hospital had wanted to go there, and 62 per cent of those in hospices.[10] On the other hand, when people who died at home were studied only 3 per cent of their relatives, looking back on it, wished the death had not been at home but in a hospital.[11] We do not know how many of our people in East London wished to die at home. We felt we could not ask them. All we can say is that, unasked, six of them were clear they wanted home.

The government also favours it. The White Paper which preceded the Community Care Act stated forthrightly that

As an increasing number of more dependent people are supported in the community there will be a need for the provision of more personal care by home care workers.[12]

It is obvious enough why this should be the official view. Carers do not have careers. It is cheaper for people to be looked after by unpaid (or partly unpaid) volunteers. There are an estimated 6 million carers in Britain, of whom 1.4 million are providing at least 20 hours of care per week either to someone living in the same household as themselves or in another household, not just to dying people but to sick people generally, the elderly and the handicapped. This volume of care would have cost between £15 billion and £24 billion if provided by paid people. Instead, it costs the state, in comparative terms, next to nothing.[13]

Why not more often?

Most of that care is not for cancer patients, although some of it is. In the long periods when they are visiting hospital only as out-patients, cancer patients are among those who need home care if they can get it. But as for dying at home, if there is in a general way a preference to die at home, why does it not happen more often? The latest available figures show that for the country as a whole the majority of people dying from cancer – 51 per cent – died in an NHS hospital.[14] Of the remainder, 18 per cent died in a hospice and 6 per cent elsewhere (mainly old people's homes), leaving only 25 per cent who died at home.

Our own enquiry – small as it was – suggests some of the reasons. Where there were no live-in carers, home was hardly an option. Where there were, dying at home was at least a choice, but only as long as the burden on the carer was not too great.[15]

The work was bound to become more wearing as the patient became more incapacitated. It could become unbearable at the end because the illness had gone on for so long. The strain of it was cumulative. For the full-time carers it could take all their time, day and night, with their sleep as much interrupted as that of the patient. They became progressively more tired. They could themselves be plagued with illnesses brought on by the strain.[16]

The carers not only had to be nurse, sometimes for patients who had become incontinent, but cook, telephonist, housekeeper and shopper all in one. Shopping trips had to be carefully organ-ised to fit in, usually early in the day when the patient felt well

enough to be left alone. After a certain stage it might be impossible to leave them at all, and someone else – if there was a
someone else – had to do the shopping. Always there was the
uncertainty of not knowing how long it would last. Inevitably,
there was a conflict in some people's minds between the wish
that the dying would never die and the wish that it would be
over. Impossible not to think sometimes about the relief that
death would bring; impossible not to feel some guilt about thinking it, or about admission to the hospice for that matter.

It was not easy to be open about the conflict. How could the
carers, even if they admitted it to themselves, say that the person
they were so deeply attached to and who they so much didn't
want to hurt would have to be sent into an institution, and,
moreover, sent by them? It could hardly fail to seem like what
dying people most fear, abandonment. Ivy had had to agree to it
at one point. Donald's medication had been changed and he was
sleeping more. One morning she could not wake him; this got
her into a state.

> I was dropping. . . . the district nurse would have to come in
> some days. I said 'Oh no. I don't want strange people coming
> in.' I was so low.

This prompted the admission to the hospice. Ivy felt a bit less
guilty because Donald's sister was with them at the time and she
confirmed that this was the right course to take.

For many carers there was the growing realisation that they
could not stand much more without cracking up themselves. This
was all the more likely because, as the illness progressed towards
its end, people were likely to become more isolated. Kenneth,
who had loved the hustle and bustle of people coming to his
home for the regular Saturday family gathering, eventually (as
we've seen) could not manage it any more. It was too tiring. He
had to ask people not to come, or to come less often. He had to
cut himself off; so his wife had been cut off too. The living room
had become even more like a sick room, as it had in the Allen's
house.

Recognising the strain on them, their GP, Dr Norgrove, had
suggested at various times that Kenneth should go into hospital,
more for Florence's sake than his own. To this Kenneth was
resolutely opposed, even when his daughters joined in and told
their father that, if the doctor said he should go into hospital, he

should: it was getting too much for their mother. Other people were more prepared to go into hospital than Kenneth; Janet and Dora did not want to be any more of a burden than they already were.

But it was the same dilemma for Dora's daughters. Their mother had been in bed at home for some weeks. The two of them, or perhaps the three of them, were getting exhausted.

> On Saturday we made the decision that mummy would go into the hospice. The Macmillan nurse said it was up to us and they would keep a bed ready there. We couldn't cope. It was physically tiring – also never knowing whether she was going to get through that day or not – we never knew. We saw her deterioration. Then she would ask for a bowl of rice pudding. She didn't die as we expected it. Even Barry[17] said 'I hope she doesn't go on much longer.' She was a very demanding person. She went into the hospice on Monday. Barry got very upset, devastated. 'It'll break her heart.'

But it didn't, or if it did, it wasn't obvious. 'She was different in the hospice, much calmer,' said one of the daughters. 'It was the drugs. I was relieved because she looked much more comfortable.' The other daughter was more upset. 'It was not someone I knew.'

It is a pity if the preference of the patient – which under favourable conditions would usually be the preference of the carer as well – cannot be met. For one thing it is only if the patient stays at home that the carer can be sure, or as sure as possible, of being there at the moment of death. The hospice Home Care service was set up in order to support home deaths, and the proportion of people dying at home would be even lower without them and their like. But the service needs more resources and, to relieve the relatives, needs to have added to it more respite places for patients. There are only a few beds for this purpose in hospices. The value of giving carers a break was shown at different times well before the end when Janet, Jennifer and Kenneth had short stays in the hospice.

Hospice or hospital?

People without live-in carers (or their equivalent) did not have the same choice between home and institution nor the stresses and comforts that such a choice brought with it. But in the last stages of their illness they did have a choice between hospital and hospice. They did not necessarily see it as a choice; often their minds were made up before they even considered alternatives. Arthur's hospital was only a long stone's throw from his home, almost as much a 'local' as his pub. It was also easier for his angel and his step-daughter to drop in there. He went there to die, without questioning it. Walter also felt he had a local hospital and took it for granted he would go there.

By contrast, Julia saw she had a choice and worried over it. She was admitted to the hospice and, several times, to the Marsden cancer hospital, including the hospital's hospice ward. She decided, eventually but unequivocally, that when comparing the two it was the hospital for her. She feared the hospice would let her fade away when she wanted, at almost all costs, to be kept alive. At the cancer hospital the crash-trolley was always ready to race to her bed if she was about 'to kick the bucket'.

Other people were as firm in their support for the hospice which Julia rejected. Jennifer was unusual as someone who had a carer at home, and yet tried out the hospice in order to get away.

I went to the hospice of my own accord because at home we were all getting on top of each other. I was getting more and more miserable and my son couldn't accept my illness. I was picking on my husband as well. I asked to go into the hospice for a couple of days for a break. I went to the chapel and spoke with the nuns and nurses and got comfort from them and from the priest who came to see me. I can't explain exactly what. It was more than just love – a form of comfort – something from inside. I said to my own priest, 'I've got something from them and I'd hate to lose it.' It's given me an inner peace. I spent three weeks there. I came home a different person.

After that Jennifer did not go back to the hospice. She died peacefully at home eight months later.[18]

Janet Rahman did not belong to the majority who thought home was best. She didn't feel cared for at home. In order to give her family a 'rest', as she put it, she admitted herself to the hospice where she was interviewed.

People here are very relaxed and understanding. They try to

make your life as comfortable as possible. I don't properly relax. I don't want fussing, just a little understanding and patience.

Here you've only got to ring the bell and someone comes. If something is worrying you, you can tell them straight away. That's important. I feel so secure. The hospice is so calming and relaxing. It's not like that at home.

The hospice was as good as it could be. Her home was not.

Dermot's hospice story was the most wonderful. He had had enough of hospitals. On the last of his many stays an infection had confined him to the single room of a special ward. He had already been impressed by the Home Care nurses so he jumped at the opportunity of the hospice when it came. When he arrived one of the sisters in the hospice did what he had never done (perhaps out of fear she would not come) and telephoned his only surviving relative, his real sister in America. She got the next plane.

In the hospice he was now surrounded with more company and fellowship than he had perhaps ever before enjoyed: other patients, his neighbour Ellen, the visiting Sisters of Charity, his sister and the co-author of this book. Seeing his sister again was

marvellous ... fantastic ... fabulous. .... It's lovely that she must have come within two days of hearing, all that way, it's really wonderful to have her here ... she comes and stays most afternoons.

I feel much calmer now ... but it's there. You know it's there all the time ... the cancer. My mind keeps turning to it ... you just don't know ... what it's going to be like. I keep thinking about it ... you don't know when.

During one of these sessions a nurse came and prepared Dermot to go and see the chiropodist. He wondered what the charge would be and was told it was all part of the service. He had never been so well cared for. He was a little worried by new symptoms that he didn't understand, particularly what he called 'the shakes' but 'the treatment here is wonderful ... they give you all the care'.

A week later his sister was with him for nearly all the hours possible. She was very upset about 'all those years lost that can't be retrieved'. Her husband, who was with her, wanted her to go back to America; but she couldn't. She couldn't sleep. While one of us was talking to Dermot, a nurse came in to say goodbye. She was off to Ireland for her holidays. Dermot bounced up in his chair to make sure she could see him saying goodbye. He relished his new wider family. Although he had been alone for so much of his life, he now embraced the community of the hospice, particularly after the isolation of barrier nursing in a special ward at the hospital.

It's not like the hospital here. There's lots going on, it's very busy, things happening all the time, giving you pills and people coming. The hospital, that was so quiet, nothing happened. I like this, I like it here.

A few days later he was sitting in the warm early morning sunshine, glasses on, reading his newspaper in his usual spot near the floor-to-ceiling window or talking with others – responding to the comradeship of other patients. He said he took communion regularly, occasionally joined by his sister. 'It helps to calm me . . . reduces the anxiety . . . about going.' He was grateful for the little details that made the hospice an emotionally warm place to be in, like Father coming round and saying good night to all the patients, cracking the odd joke. He was finding it easier to talk with his sister now they had built bridges across the time-gap. 'All those years . . . I regret losing all those years. It was my fault that we didn't keep in touch.' He was more relaxed, but still

troubled about the cancer, you know, when it will be, and how. They can't tell you, give you a date or time. You don't know. My sister says that you must live from day to day but it's difficult.

Two weeks into February his sister spent the whole day at his bedside. Her view was 'we must live today, yesterday has gone'. Dermot sat at the end of the short ward in a wing back chair by the window, upright, as always, without the support of pillows, reading his paper. He could no longer manage books. They required too much concentration. It was Valentine's Day and his sister had sent him an affectionate card. He had a slight cold and cough which troubled him so he hadn't had his daily bath.

A week later it was raining with no morning sunshine. Dermot was again sitting in his chair as straight as his frailty would allow. He was weak and unsteady but didn't like the idea of bed. He was never a bed person. His sister had arrived early with his daily newspaper. He was tired and talked and moved very little.

Four days later he died and was flown by his sister and her husband to his home village in Ireland to be buried next to his mother and father.

* * *

The Allens, the Chandlers and the Barnes as presented in the first part of this chapter were closer to the traditional family than any others amongst our people, except the Knights. They had children, their children had children and they had remained in close touch; and, partly because their extended families had kept them busy and satisfied in a respected role, the wives had been the opposite of career women. Perhaps it was no accident that the two husbands lasted so much longer than their doctors had expected, and, despite all their disabilities, had made so much of their extra time. Having a wife, a husband or a close partner to look after you, and children to help, is the best state.

But the auguries for that kind of family are not all that favourable. On present trends there are likely to be less Allens, Chandlers, Knights and Barnes in the future. Unless countervailing tendencies develop, dying is going to be more miserable in the twenty-first century. Medicine will be that much more sophisticated than the medicine of this century, keeping people alive longer; lingering illnesses could as a result become even more common while the setting in which people linger becomes less and less desirable, especially for older widowed people who cannot be cared for by a spouse. One survey suggested that 'The consequence of all this is that the very old were more likely to be cared for by people who, in retrospect, felt that it would have been better if the old person had died earlier.'[19]

It would, of course, be a boon if the health and the life expectancy of men could be improved. Men who die first are in one way lucky: they more often have someone to look after them. But if men lived as long as women – or, on average, if as many husbands survived their wives as wives survive their husbands – it could represent a kind of gender equality adding significantly to human happiness. Widows would be less common, men better off because they would live longer, and more women better off because they would be looked after when they were ill and dying. There would be an all-round gain.

It would be an offset to the great trends of this century – the decline in fertility which has reduced the number of children able to help ailing parents, the geographical dispersal of the family, and, above all, its increasing fragility. People who had preserved and nurtured their marriages had a resource which could go far towards sustaining them through the crisis. Where the parents had stayed together, the children had not been required to take sides between mother and father. But at least for the time being this kind of family support is on the wane.

Yet we were surprised that the patients living alone, while on that account less fortunate, managed so well. Most of the children of marriages broken by separation or death did not desert their parents. They responded when their father or mother was in such critical need. Death could be a healing force as well as a destructive one. Close friends were not so much in evidence except for Julia's friend Maria, but the healing effect of death seemed to work for neighbours as well as relatives.

We had expected that when close relatives were not available, in an emergency, other kin would do something to fill the gap. That belongs to the common pattern of family life, not just in Britain. The substitutions may not occur as smoothly as they once did for dependent children or the dependent elderly or the dependent dying; but family bonds are still strong enough to be felt as duties. Ties which would in normal times be almost forgotten are activated when needs are laid bare by death.

What we did not expect – and this is perhaps the most striking conclusion of the chapter – was that the imminence of death could bring out the same kind of solidarity amongst neighbours. Ellen behaved as 'if she was a sister'; Myra likewise; Maria was closer than that. They could not be said to have a duty of any ordinary kind, through the discharge of which they would incur some right to repayment by someone else with a reciprocal duty. Performing such a duty is, amongst other things, a matter of self-interest even in the family, if there is the hope of some return. Neighbours do not have such a duty, and cannot assert any claim to a return for their generosity. Their actions belong more to altruism than duty. Such unselfishness is a continuation of what used to be ordinary neighbourliness in this district. But as well as that, death is not only an extraordinary event for the dying but brings out extraordinary behaviour in other people. In face of the common threat, it seems as much an expression of the solidarity of humanity as of the family.

Whether it is family or people who behave like family when they are not, what stands out is the lengths to which carers were prepared to go. They were under continuous and long-drawn-out strain themselves, working hard to keep body and soul as much together as possible, watching the deterioration, the accelerated ageing of someone with whom they identified, fearing the pain of abandonment which death would bring to them. Why did they do it? They were much more than volunteers, although they were of course also that. They worked as hard as any person being paid a wage. Where the carers were spouses or children, and the family had been a loving one, they had that to sustain them – the attachments of a lifetime and the shared memories, of marriages and births and other deaths, of strange uncles and loving aunts, of trips together, of adversities borne in common. The commitment of caring also unfolds and builds on itself. Once the carer has started on the task, a momentum builds up. The close intimacy between carer and cared for generates its own feelings which both take the place of, and reinforce, obligation. There can also be something very special and love-inspiring about the imminence of death. Death can bring out life-giving qualities.

> The far most fulfilling months of my life, probably, were when at the age of 33 I was co-ordinating care for my neighbour (a single lady in her sixties) who was dying of cancer. There is something inherently meaningful, it seems to me, about caring for a dying person, as indeed there is about caring for young children.[20]

However people were sustained, and even have a sense of themselves 'growing' through the intensity of their experience, there could be no disguising the strain, nor the need for the unpaid (unless paid with gratitude) to be supported by the paid. In modern conditions, and with modern knowledge of palliative medicine, the carers need to be cared for by specialists who visit the home.

In other words they need a home nursing service of the kind which in this part of East London is so well developed and should be equally so all over the country. It embodies the right idea – back-up for the patient and carers, whoever they may be. There are other variants on the same model, and we mention some of

these, at such places as Paddington, Doncaster, Peterborough and
Lambeth, in Appendix II.

Home nursing services, driven in part by the need to reduce
spending on hospitals, could offset our gloomy prognosis about
the effects on home care of changes in the family. When home
nursing expands, as it should do, more people may be able to
achieve their aim of dying at home. More families, however much
shredded by the advances of an individualistic and restless society,
may then be able to do more for their dying relatives, even
though it would be hard to surpass the dedication of a Lilian or
a Florence. The understanding could be that the home nursing
teams of the future could do their part to back up relatives and
neighbours. Formality will then underpin the informal, and duty
nurture altruism, in a compact appropriate to the solemnity of
death.

Chapter 5

The doctor

So far we have said rather little, except in passing, about doctors and their relationships with the patients. This is a crucial matter which can be delayed no longer. Doctors must now be brought into the centre of the scene on which they have such a profound effect. Modern science and technology have given them a pre-eminence in the struggle against death.

The pre-eminence is relatively new. Many of the infectious diseases, like cholera, smallpox, tuberculosis, diptheria, measles and scarlet fever, which used to be the great killers have been overcome, not so much by curing people when they are ill as by preventing them from becoming ill. The role of medicine has become ever more important as the infectious and contagious diseases have given way to the non-infectious diseases which are as yet so much less amenable to prevention by means of environmental control.

Doctors and their allies have now for the time being become responsible for the thrust of modern civilisation towards greater and more sophisticated control over life. Doctors also seem to be more obviously the controllers because they deal on an individual basis with individual people who call on them for help, whereas the agriculturalists who produce more food and the engineers who deliver cleaner water (if they can hold off the effects of environmental contamination) exert their preservative power unseen and in the large. Compared to them, nothing could be less remote and more horribly personal than a surgeon who slices into your most vital organs with knife or laser. Doctors seem to have the power which used to be the preserve of the priest: as sometimes overstated, the power of life and death.

Their power derives from a new but already ingrained habit of mind which they share with their patients. Both know that death is the inescapable lot of human beings, but still death is viewed as the result of a cause, or causes, which can be pinned down and, once the cause is understood, becomes preventable, or more preventable. Law and practice fosters this near-omnipotent attitude by requiring doctors, when filling out death certificates, to state the cause. As if age will not find us all out in the end when the internal machinery runs down, 'old age' or 'insufficient will to live' will not do as a cause, but cancer of this or that sort or a coronary of this or that sort will pass muster and be put into its proper slot in the national table of mortality. One far-sighted surgeon admitted that 'In thirty-five years as a licensed physician, I have never had the temerity to write "Old Age" on a death certificate, knowing that the form would be returned to me with a terse note from some official record-keeper informing me that I had broken the law. Everywhere in the world, it is illegal to die of old age.'[1]

Putting a name to a cause is itself a step towards control – grist alike for the epidemiological researcher and for the patient who can find satisfaction in saying that he or she is suffering from . . . . Even if the name is in the Greek or Latin which doctors still employ, rolling it around your tongue can become a kind of magic which suggests at once that the doctors know what they are doing and may be able to do for you. Where there's a cause, there's hope. For the doctor, identification of a cause is the vital precursor to treatment which may prolong life, while scientists and technologists behind them are chasing the contributory array of causes behind the overall cause as labelled and, by gaining more knowledge about the underlying mechanisms, trying to develop yet further improvements in treatment, and further extensions to life. The belief that death always has a cause, and if understood may be avertible, buttresses the overriding ethic of doctors, which is to hold death at bay. Death when it comes is a defeat, but in a battle not a war. The medicines can still seem like elixirs of life, and newspapers, playing on a wishful gullibility, can repeatedly proclaim a cure for cancer for people not born to die but to attend the out-patient clinic.

The cast of mind proper to the heroic undertaking is a pervasive hopefulness which sustains a great range of health cults from jogging to the most punishing forms of dieting. Samuel Johnson said, 'Hope is itself a species of happiness, and, perhaps, the chief happiness which this world affords',[2] especially, he might have said, in the sickroom. The duty of doctors is to keep hope alive, and thence to keep intact the presumption that death can be held off for at least a bit longer. In our technological society we are supposed to live, not to die – which means that to die with equanimity is all the more of an achievement for an individual who the general culture can, when no hope is left, callously leave to fend for himself or herself.[3]

Hustle and bustle

The doctor can be an awesomely knowing figure. But this is not necessarily how the patients see them in the setting in which doctors (and nurses, of course) often have to operate. Not the carpeted rooms of the private wing; no private phones for the patients to keep in touch with home; no knocking on doors to ask for permission to enter. But hospital wards, which are sometimes like Clapham Junction in the rush hour, with doctors in white coats and solemn faces moving around continuously between their platforms, nurses dashing from one bed to another, cleaners with mops, porters pushing unconscious people on trolleys and trying not to get the drips snarled up. This is the setting in which life-and-death communication has to insert itself.

There may not even be time for any communication when so much has to be done in the general rush. Jack Dickson could not empty his bladder. This took him to hospital and the hospital took to him, controlling the painful and alarming symptom, and keeping him in thereafter until he could feed himself after the treatment. On one busy day, that is one normal day, except not normal for him, a nursing sister arrived at his bed with his tray for lunch and, since she thought he was not capable of acting for himself, she fed him. He could not chew or swallow at the rate he was being plied with food by her. The next mouthful was pushed into his mouth before the last one had disappeared. He tried to hold off the dreadful spoon and to complain to her before his mouth was gagged up again with food he could not swallow. She could not listen, or at any rate did not. The ward clock was ticking away. Lunch had to be cleared before the visitors flocked in at 2 o'clock. Jack could not get it down in time, and could not explain. His sister came in at 2. He said to her (not of course to the nursing sister): 'They're trying to murder me in here.' His sister looked at him as blankly as the nurse. She had three other relatives to visit in hospital. She was busy too. She changed the subject of conversation and asked, instead, where he kept all his money now he wasn't spending it. 'Under the bed?' she queried.

The patients we saw were very few and yet they could not be understood except in a more general context. They are amongst the millions of patients treated every year in the NHS and so are caught up in any change in the general standards and implicit codes of behaviour of the doctors and others. In order to gauge what the patients said the first necessity is to take account of their individual temperament and individual experience; but they were also all dealing with doctors whose collective behaviour has as a body been altering, with enormous variations between them, but all the same with a certain pattern. The practice of 'telling all' has, for instance, been changing rapidly.

Quite apart from his or her busyness, the problematic nature of the doctor's crucial role as a communicator can be brought out by referring to some general features of the relations between consumers and producers. Producers almost always know more about their product than the buyers, and in their selling they have an interest (which of course they can resist) in concealing, or playing down, any weaknesses it has, and exaggerating, or playing up, its virtues. If the product is complex the buyers are liable to be ignorant, gullible and exploitable, and can suffer repeatedly from the unequal relationship. Hence the consumer movement which has grown up in this century. It has had some small success in requiring or persuading producers to be more truthful in the information they give to consumers so that they can make more sensible choices when they buy one product or service rather than another. The advances of 'consumerism' have also had some influence upon medical practice.

But doctors are not ordinary suppliers. If they were judged by the same standards, in the past hardly one of them would have escaped being taken to court at some time for misinformation or misrepresentation. The relationship is different from that of ordinary suppliers and consumers in many ways. For one thing, the knowledge differential is so much more pronounced. Though many lay people are better informed nowadays, the ignorance of lay people about the way their bodies work is still astonishing, despite the thriving health cults and the abundance of articles about health in newspapers and magazines, on programmes on radio and television. But for children who do not take biology as a subject at school, there is still almost no systematic health education. So doctors know a great deal more about you, at any rate about one rather vital component of you, your body, than you do yourself. If told you have cancer in a particular organ you may be more confused about where your organ is, and even more what its function is, than you are about the nature of the cancer which is attacking it. If you were ever asked to point to your pancreas or your gall bladder or your hippocampus or pineal gland, would you know where to point? Would you know the function of your liver, your lymphatic system or your circadian clocks which govern and orchestrate your array of bodily rhythms?

Doctors know they have such intimate insight into you because, within limits, your body works in the same way as anyone else's. One of the authors of this book asked the surgeon who cut away part of his colon whether the surgeon would be able to recognise his insides if he ever had the misfortune to reveal them to him again, incognito, and he answered emphatically no. In the absence of gross pathology, a president or prince looks much like the more humble of us, on the inside, although on the surface, and in our minds, we are as different as our fingerprints or our handwriting, often even more extravagantly so. But hidden from ordinary view, we are almost as alike as the products which come off the conveyor belt of a mass-production system, and it is this which gives a doctor his power. He can be trained on Mr X and cut up Mrs Y.

So if it were only the alikeness of our insides that mattered, the information which had to be given to patients by doctors could be as closely prescribed as for any product. There would be nothing to stop governments requiring doctors to tell all, or a good deal, when they proposed to remove or repair the standard organs of a standard patient. The knowledge gap is so large and the service often is so much more crucial than anything else the consumer ever has need of that the case for such a requirement could be far stronger than for ordinary services.

It cannot be. The doctor may understand the body of his patient in a general way but it does not follow that he or she positively knows what is wrong with it, and certainly does not know what exactly the outcome of the treatment will be. The ignorance of the patient is also too great. If he or she were to understand it all, an intensive training would have to be given to every patient before treatment could begin, beyond what they could get from broadcast programmes, articles in the press and popular books. Every patient would have to start by being a student. As it is, the doctor or nurse has to explain on the only assumption that can ordinarily be made, that the patient knows little or nothing. The doctor has had a hard enough job understanding it in the language of science, and even then may well not be sure about it, and certainly not sure whether the treatment will be effective, and yet has to explain it in the language of the street or – more demanding even than that – in the languages of many different streets and of many different lay people with varying amounts of education and familiarity with complex ways of thinking and talking. A modern man of science is called upon to explain what he thinks is going on inside the body of the patient opposite him when behind the beseeching eyes looking out at him may be all manner of strange ideas which hark back to medieval times and before, with magic and superstition not far from the surface. It is easy for the knowledgeable to feel superior, even impatient with the patient; when the mind opposite seems so inscrutable, or confused, it is easy to treat the body as if there was no mind within it anxiously fumbling about trying to understand what is happening.

So whatever information there is has to be tailored to the person. This is why any general regulation needs to be hedged about. The NHS Management Executive Handbook has this to say in its *Guide to Consent for Examination on Treatment 1991:*

> Patients are entitled to receive sufficient information in a way that they can understand about the proposed treatments, the possible alternatives and any substantial risks, so that they can make a balanced judgement.[4]

'In a way that they can understand' – the doctor has to make a judgement about that and the patient's judgement about the doctor often follows on. The knower circles the unknower and the unknower the knower. Or the person in the white coat may have done it so many times before that the explanation, so far as it is given at all, comes more by rote than it does from an attempt to understand what is in the patient's mind.

Wise doctors, who are not just rote doctors doing what has always been done before, have therefore to try to gauge how much a patient is capable of taking in at the first diagnosis, and at every subsequent stage when there is a check-up or some new treatment is started or some new symptom explained.[5] Other things being equal, they will err on the side of saying too much if they know of the research which has been done suggesting that patients – even children – have better rates of recovery or pain relief when they are given a lot of information about their condition and treatment.[6]

The doctor cannot bank on patients just ignoring facts they do not want to know, adept as patients (and all other people) are at censoring out disagreeable information. Mrs Anstey, for instance, did not want to know, or to know much. She would say 'I've cancer you know' in a wondering sort of way, and then show she did not know what it was or what it could do. She fastened on the word rather than the disease.

But they may not always be able to act as their own censor when the doctor is facing them across the table and trying to make them understand what they learned about an ailment from their auntie when they were this high is just wrong. The auntie is not there; the doctor is, and even though he or she never had any training in how to communicate with lay people, what is said may sometimes be so persuasive that the new information will overcome all the mental barricades that are raised against it and lodge painfully in a mind that would (for its own good reasons) much rather not be its host. Morale may plummet as a result. So the doctor needs to make a judgement about that rather than taking it for granted that the unwanted will be unheeded.

Jack Dickson, one of our oldest people, was a case in point. He was content enough with doctors who summed him up for what he was, a born-and-bred cockney and proud of it. If they assumed he would therefore be the sort of person who would not want to know in any detail, or even in broad outline, about his illness, and would rather not make any decisions but place himself almost unreservedly, calmly and without fuss, in the doctor's hands (metaphorically as well as literally), then they were right. Just before we first saw him he had been in hospital 'under radar treatment'. 'I had it every day. They tried to burn it out of me for 28 days. Then they discharged me.' It was all very matter of fact. On a previous occasion he caught an infection after his major operation and had four or five minor operations afterwards 'because it wouldn't heal up'. He ended up with a colostomy bag for the rest of his life. 'There were no explanations.' 'But I've had too many operations in the past to worry. I never worried.'

Unlike some others, he was not put out when the doctor he expected to see in the hospital – his usual doctor – was not the one he saw, or when a locum turned up instead of his own GP. He had had the shakes a few nights previously and his neighbour had phoned the GP.

> He was a stand-in. He gave me some tablets for it. I don't mind about seeing different doctors all the time. I just leave it to them. There's nothing else to do is there?

He wanted the doctor to be in total command. As long as there are patients like him, doctors will have good reason for not going overboard to tell all.

How then are doctors to know how much of Jack there is in the patient sitting in front of them? Hunch? That will be part of it. But less chancey tactics are now being used as well. At the Royal London Hospital and elsewhere it has, for instance, been found useful to ask patients a general question before the consultation. Dr Fallowfield has conducted a research project on this issue. Researchers asked cancer patients before they saw the doctor

a) if they wanted all information whether good or bad;
b) if they wanted information only if it is good;
c) if they wanted to leave it up to the doctor.

Ninety-five per cent of people fell into category (a), 3 per cent into (b) and 2 per cent into (c).[7]

The search is on for good practice. One can reasonably hope that in time the relationship between the more knowledgeable and the more ignorant will become more of a partnership, and a partnership which leans towards the patient rather than the doctor, putting the patient as much in command as possible, and which leans, also, towards preventive rather than curative medicine. Popularising without bowdlerising or patronising may turn out to be the great advance in medicine in the next century, putting penicillin and the other wonder-drugs in the shade. In that next stage of medicine, treatment by the word may become as significant as treatment by the scalpel or drugs. An American doctor referred to it in those terms in his advice to his colleagues. 'But try to do as little harm as possible, not only in treatment with drugs, or with the knife, but also in treatment with words, with the expression of your sentiments and emotions.'[8] One could add glances, demeanours, gestures. They can all kill or cure. The heedless doctor 'is inflicting a wound upon the recipient's psyche as surely as he would be inflicting one on the individual's soma should he incise his or her abdomen – but here it is without the benefit of anesthesia.'[9]

A new relationship will not happen without squaring up to the problematic nature of the relationship. The expert on one side of the table or above the bed knows both how much more he or she knows than the patient about the relatively hard facts of diagnosis and the less hard facts about the prognosis. On the other side, or way below, is the patient who could be without the most complex organism which has yet emerged from billions of years of evolution for all the patient knows about what he or she *is*. But if one were to accept that the marvellous creation belongs to the expert rather than to the layperson it would be to prescribe a regime of autocracy for all sick people. Democracy would only be for the healthy, and the ghost would be given up. All that can properly be done is to move on, and, allowing for the differences, to make the situation of the medical consumer first as good as that of ordinary consumers, and then better. To each person his own cancer, to each cancer its own person. The same goes for any other malfunctioning of our internal machinery which is, though common to all of us, so intricate that not even the greatest expert yet understands more than a little about it.

A quiet revolution

The changes at present afoot show there are grounds for hope. It appears that in the second half of the century more doctors have become more informative with their patients, or at least believe that they should be so in dealing with the dying, despite the fact that medicine has become ever more specialised and technical and so more difficult to explain. In the new mental climate doctors are having to face up more explicitly to the dilemma we have touched on of how best to tell their patients without undermining their morale.

The latest turn follows on a long period in which there was little openness. According to Ariès, 'The beginning of the lie', as he called it, began in the middle of the nineteenth century when

a long-standing frankness was abandoned.[10] Gorer says that even
in the late nineteenth century 'death was no mystery, except in
the sense that death is always a mystery'.[11] But there is a measure
of agreement that at some point death was driven into secrecy.
It was concealed by confining the dying in hospitals, and by the
corporate solidarity and structural blindness of doctors for whom
death was (and still is) a failure. It was not until the late 1950s
that another change set in, and, partly due to improved therapies,
and the greater optimism amongst doctors, the older more traditional frankness was restored in a new form.

Wouters, in a well-known paper, has a different chronology but
his account of what happened in Holland in the period of what
he called 'the sacred lie' was very similar. The motives for lying
were no less high than they are today for not lying – to prevent
mental suffering – the difference being that then it was thought
that the best way to prevent it was to leave patients in the dark
so that they could believe (even against the evidence of their
bodies) that they would get better;[12] whereas today it is increasingly thought that the best way to prevent suffering is to tell
people what is wrong and what is going to be done to help them,
and why. Up to the 1950s Dutch courage used to be maintained
by lying.

> Where there's life, there's hope, and in order to preserve hope,
> every physician allowed for a 'pia fraus' (sacred lie) when
> dealing with the gravest cases, where the patient was dying.[13]

The switchover to greater openness seems to have come later
in Britain. According to Cartwright and Anderson,[14] in 1969 the
practice was not so very different from what it had been in
Holland. But by the time a repeat study was made by Seale
in 1987 the new vogue had taken hold:

> The results from professionals suggest a general preference for
> openness about illness and death, tempered by the consider-
> ation that bad news needs to be broken slowly, in a context
> of support, while recognising that not everyone wishes to know
> all.
>
> Results suggest that there has been a trend towards greater
> openness about diagnosis and death between doctors and
> patients, and this has been particularly marked in the case of
> hospital doctors and cancer patients.[15]

In this change the growth of the hospice movement has played
an important part, along with changes in the pattern of mortal
illness – and particularly the increased incidence of slow death
like that from cancer. Cicely Saunders, the founder of the
extremely influential St Christopher's Hospice in South London,
has been the great pioneer. She combined the methods of allevia-
tory dosing to deal with pain which had been developed at St
Luke's Hospital and the religious tradition of openness which
had characterised the St Joseph's Hospice, which was the base
for our enquiry. Rory Williams has attributed the differences in
attitude between one part of the country and another to the
variable diffusion of hospices.

> Thus Aberdeen, at a time when it had no hospice, and in a
> geographical position in north-east Scotland which was rela-
> tively isolated, continued to conserve attitudes mostly typical
> of an earlier period of silence and avoidance.[16]

This, while in London the change in attitudes was well under
way.

Parallel changes in the US

There have been the same sort of changes in the US. In 1961
Oken[17] found that 88 per cent of responding physicians preferred
not to tell a cancer patient his diagnosis. By 1977, according to
Novack, there had been a complete reversal, with 98 per cent
indicating a preference the other way. The new behaviour, like the
old, was 'supported by strong belief and emotional involvement in
its being right'.

> The rise in the consumerism movement and increasing public
> scrutiny of the medical profession have altered the physician–
> patient relationship. In this era of 'patients' rights', an attitude
> of frankness feels right and, indeed, given the current dispu-
> tatious atmosphere of medical practice, may be the safest one
> to adopt.[18]

In the long period when the lie was whiter than white, patients
must often have known full well the truth was withheld, but,
unless they had exceptional confidence, they could not challenge
their doctor to come out with it. Now that the convention has
swung around, instances abound, and are made public, of the

futility of trying to conceal what is often obvious. Patients find out. They talk to other patients. They pick up small signs. Kenneth Chandler noticed that

> there were no drugs for me and the alarm bells did ring. The doctor said 'see you in two weeks' and everyone else was coming back in two months. They said 'Professor Bennett is coming to see you', and then I knew in myself.

A look can be enough, an evasiveness, a show of embarrassment. The hospital can inadvertently give the game away. One man interviewed for another survey was not told by his GP anything about the possibility of his having cancer when he referred him to a consultant in the hospital. A few weeks later the man received the notification of an appointment from the 'Oncology Department', a name which can for the layperson itself represent a concealment. But he was curious enough to go to his local library to consult a dictionary and there found that in practice oncology meant cancer. He was thrown into a distress from which he did not wholly recover. He remained suspicious of doctors thereafter. It showed how painful the truth can be when it is stumbled upon. If a fact about yourself which could hardly be more important has been concealed from you and you find out, it can set off a general distrust about everything you are told, or not told, from that point on. It can certainly undermine the confidence which a patient has in the doctor.

Glaser and Strauss,[19] in a study made in the 1960s (before the change had taken hold) which has not yet become totally irrelevant, called one reaction 'suspected awareness' ('the situation where the patient suspects what the other knows and therefore attempts to confirm or invalidate the suspicion'). This can absorb the patient, making him or her warily look out for any hint to help the patient to decide for themself. Or it can, perhaps more usually, produce a similar but even more confused and debilitating state of 'mutual pretence awareness' ('the situation where each party defines the patient as dying, but each pretends that the other has not done so'). People can die squeezed into a double lie which can sour their relationships with doctors and nurses just at the time when they most need to be able to talk frankly about their fears and worries, and need others to be frank with them. To be surrounded by deceptive bromides is exactly what most people do not want. 'How can he gain the ease of wholly sincere talk with others if all maintain the pretence that his imminent departure from life, his leaving them for ever, is just not taking place?'[20] The train is just about to reach its destination and the passenger is the only person who is supposed not to know.

How in such a case can they set their affairs in order, make a will, avoid starting a business or any venture which they will not be able to complete? How can they try to moderate damage they may have done to others, take stock of their lives or rediscover, or discover, their religion, if that is what they would want to do? How can they give consent to the treatment they are having if the doctors do not give them all the information they need in order to come to a decision? They may have terrible fears about what is going to happen which could be allayed only if they could be voiced. Before the change in opinion had set in, Cicely Saunders put the point well in a comment made in 1965 on a patient who 'overheard' her diagnosis.

> How do we feel about those who discover it in such ways, unable because officially they do not 'know' to hear of good hopes of cure, of palliation, of the unlikelihood of distress for them or of possibilities of help should it occur.[21]

It matters so much because it is only if they have information that people will be able to maintain some control over what remains of their lives. In this context as in so many others information is power. It also matters a great deal to the carers. It has been shown that their misery, when they have become survivors, can be somewhat alleviated if they have had frank forewarning, and been able to prepare themselves in their minds for what is to come.

Mutual reinforcement

The freeing up of information is one of four more or less distinguishable though interlinked changes which have reinforced each other. We leave aside the influence of 'consumerism'. Information apart, the first is that, as we have said before, cancer has become more treatable. The diagnosis is no longer a death sentence to be summarily executed. There is now some hope, some prospect of a better outcome to talk about and a longer period of remission. In the past the diagnosis could be concealed the more effectively because there was a relatively short period before the end. Now that life for many has been prolonged, and people return to hospitals time and again and may undergo many different kinds of treatment in the course of their illness, it has become well nigh impossible to hide the truth except from patients who are determined to hide it from themselves. The prolongation of life has certainly had the effect of making people more frank about the disease.

Second is the growth of the hospice movement. In a different setting from hospitals, different ideas can flourish. The main purpose of a hospital is to cure, not look after people who are beyond cure, and too often people die on busy acute wards. Nurses sometimes have no time to talk to patients who are largely beyond their help. Communication can be poor with and between staff,[22] poor too the control of pain mentioned in the next chapter, treatment superfluous,[23] privacy and space lacking for the family to be with the dying.[24]

But hospices are not for cure: they are for care. Palliative medicine takes over when alleviation is all that is possible. The 'sacred honesty' for which hospices stand has benefited others who are not so ill as our own patients,[25] just as greater honesty with cancer patients has in its turn benefited people suffering from quite different diseases. The pioneers have stated the principles in ways which give them a much larger relevance. Here is Parkes again.

If only the patient and the family can be helped to share the truth instead of avoiding it, the general level of tension will often be reduced and the need for drugs to reduce emotional tension artificially will diminish. Unfortunately, doctors and nurses usually find it easier to administer the drugs than to take the time to talk with patients and family members in the hope of resolving rather than repressing their problems.[26]

As we said in the introduction, the people in our study were all being visited from a hospice by Home Care nurses – Macmillan nurses as our informants almost always called them. This alone meant there could no longer be any concealment about what they were suffering from. These nurses set a standard by which others could be judged. 'With the doctors,' said Donald Knight, 'you're just a number but with Macmillan they treat me as an individual person.'

But the nurses can also be terrifying. One of his daughters said of Jack Dickson, despite his being so willing to put himself in the hands of doctors, that: 'He wouldn't consider the hospice. He thinks as soon as you go in there you're dead. You don't come out.' Kenneth Chandler likewise: 'East Enders are generally very afraid of them. They say "get there and within a fortnight you've gone from this world".' For them it was a matter of 'Abandon hope all ye that enter here.' Bringing a nursing team into a home was sometimes shied away from for the same reason. 'I always thought I wouldn't have those people near me.'

A third stream of influence has come from the United States. The law is different there, allowing (according to a general view amongst British doctors, too readily allowing) aggrieved patients to take legal action against their physicians, especially where there is some doubt whether or not consent for a particular procedure has been given. To reduce malpractice claims, doctors are required by their insurers to spell out, in what to most British patients would be considered far too much detail, the treatments they are consenting to, and their possible consequences. Doctors have to tell much more than would be considered 'all' in Britain. But the example has not been lost on British doctors.

One of the foremost proponents of openness is Dr Kübler-Ross who we mentioned earlier. She has shown that many dying people and their relatives need the opportunity, and the encouragement, to talk about the state they are in. Patients and their families may know quite well that death is imminent, and yet not say anything about it. They can easily believe that by staying silent they can protect each other from a truth that is all the more deadly for being inescapable. But if they can be encouraged to put such well-meant reticence aside, it can be an enormous relief.

> Those who have the strength and the love to sit with a dying patient in the *silence that goes beyond words* will know that this moment is neither frightening nor painful, but a peaceful cessation of the functioning of the body.[27]

Britain has followed America.

> The general philosophy of how physicians talk to cancer patients in this country has changed dramatically over the last 20 years. In the 1960s, most doctors did not reveal the true diagnosis to their patients. Instead, a full and frank discussion

was held with a close family member and a conspiracy of silence was maintained. This changed in the early 1970s when a much franker approach came from across the Atlantic. In the USA the frankness was carried to an almost brutal extreme.[28]

In course of transition

Yet we must not exaggerate. Our patients and the doctors we heard about at second hand from them were caught up in the transition. Some doctors (even some older ones who got no whiff of the new practice in their own training as medical students) have wholeheartedly embraced the new openness; others have barely been touched by it. A study of the practice of hospital doctors was made not long ago by Dr Davey.[29]

The doctors in Davey's enquiry were ready enough to tell patients they had suffered a heart attack or heart failure. But about cancer they were reluctant. One group of doctors, mainly surgeons, assumed that patients would not want to know: they were unwilling to reveal the diagnosis unless the patients asked directly, and even then they covered up by giving a much more positive prognosis than the diagnosis warranted. Their tactic depended on the patient's age, accent, vocabulary and air of confidence. The doctors' attitude was described as that of 'benevolent paternalism'. They thought that, if the patient did not ask, it was generally safe to assume that he or she did not want to know – and this must be especially so if the patient was elderly, working class and poorly educated. The other group of doctors, mainly physicians, leant the other way, believing not that they should hold back unless asked to tell but that they should tell unless asked not to. They had an attitude of what was called 'pragmatic openness'. They believed it unethical to conceal information from a patient without compelling reason. The first group of doctors believed that unsolicited bad news caused unnecessary anguish or would destroy a fighting spirit,[30] whereas the others considered that the initial distress on being told the truth was preferable to the prolonged anxiety and confusion caused by ambiguity.

A more recent study of junior doctors and nurses in a London teaching hospital has produced much the same results.[31] All of them said there had been a move towards more open communication, but no training in how to go about it, either when having to tell relatives about a sudden death or about a fatal illness. It could be particularly trying for a young doctor dealing with an old person, old enough to be his or her grandparent.

It was quite bad in my first year as a House Officer. There were a few times when I was on my own from the word go. It was very, very difficult. I had to work on my own without any guidelines. I found myself having to face relatives and not know what to say or what to do.

Another doctor said it was very difficult for any of them to see death through the eyes of relatives. 'They have been involved with death their whole career, which started with dissecting dead bodies.' Hardened themselves, often they did not want to face people who were not. Yet another doctor said:

There is a chicken way of doing it on the ward round, and not giving someone adequate time to speak to you, because time is precious to you. Does that sound callous?

Whatever the professionals do or do not do, it is unlikely to be challenged by patients who are ill and therefore preoccupied and usually lacking in confidence. In a hospital the obvious thing to do is to follow the lead given by the doctor. If he or she is close-lipped, giving no more information than seems absolutely essential, the ordinary docile patient is going to assume it is better not to ask. They are not going to risk upsetting someone in whose hands they have placed their life. If they are not going to get much information then, to avoid disappointment, the best thing is not to want it. People's expectations of each other are the ground of their behaviour, particularly when at least on one side there is uncertainty about how to behave. One kind of doctor tells little because he or she thinks that is what the patient wants (or at any rate should want) and the patient asks little because he or she thinks that is what the doctor wants.

If doctors are reticent, there can be a knock-on effect on nurses. They can be in a particularly uncomfortable position when they are not supposed to say anything which goes against what the doctor has said. Dr Davey made another study of nurses. Nurses report (he said) that some doctors too often evade cancer patients' questions or use ambiguous language and that most forget to inform nurses about what has been said to patients about their diagnosis and prognosis. Doctors and nurses agree that patients are more likely to discuss their anxieties with nurses and to ask nurses for clarification if a doctor has used an ambiguous term. However most, but not all, doctors consider nurses to be insufficiently trained or intellectually inadequate or too afraid of responsiblity to answer these questions accurately and therefore prefer nurses to be evasive, even if they have to tell white lies.[32]

So the trend towards more openness has not yet embraced the whole of the medical profession by any means. It has been uneven. The wrong people are still sometimes told the bad news; they can be more precise about the time left to a patient than they should be. A lot of the things that go wrong are the result of doctors not having enough time to talk to patients. While fully acknowledging how very difficult it is to find the right line between telling too much and telling too little, we will consider three of the common failings in turn.

Telling the wrong person first

In one crucial respect there may not yet be anything like consensus in the medical profession. More doctors are more open about cancer (and other diseases) – we do not doubt that is so, despite the uneven spread. But with whom? Not necessarily with the patient or, if with the patient, they may give a more optimistic view to him or her than to the relatives. Seale found that

> The general picture ... is that of professionals in this field preferring open communication with patients and their relatives. However, telling relatives first was the most common strategy advocated in both 1969 and 1987.[33]

Doctors thereby saved themselves the stress of having to impart bad news face to face. But they did this only at a cost, sometimes a very heavy cost, to the patients. Amongst our people, the Knights showed how unfortunate the practice could be.

The Knights had a long-lasting marriage. Some of their relatives said that Ivy had 'coddled' Donald. But despite her natural inclination they had not been able to talk together about his illness. This was the doctor's doing. He had not told Donald anything direct although before the operation Donald had made a point of asking that he should be told afterwards what the outcome was. All he and Ivy were told to begin with was that he was being referred to the Macmillan service. Ivy, never having heard of it, asked what it was. The doctor then called Ivy out from the bedside into the hospital corridor, thronged with people, and said, brusquely, without giving her the chance to ask anything or say anything, that her husband had cancer. 'He's got cancer. I've got to go now', looking at his watch. He dashed away, leaving Ivy alone, stunned and unsure whether to return to the ward and tell her husband. Understandably, she decided against this.

The doctor was not so unusual. He may have been afraid, like many others, that the patient would blame 'them personally for the bad news that they bring',[34] and that the patient would be more likely to burst out angrily at him than a relative. But he was passing the responsibility to someone who did not know what to do with the dreaded information. Does the fact that the doctor will not tell the patient directly mean that he thinks the patient should not be (perhaps could not stand being) told? Is the more or less implicit advice to the relative to keep silent?

If that is what the relative does, it means that he or she has to lie to the patient from that time on, and about a topic which is frequently on both their minds. The lie can create collusion right up to death, the patient wondering what the doctor has said, or what else the doctor has said if something is known, or even knowing full well what the doctor has said but unable to challenge the relative because no information has been volunteered, and the relative cannot be caught out in a lie. On the side of the relative, once he or she has lied at all by not passing on right away what the doctor has said, it becomes ever more difficult to return to it. Come out with it a month later and the patient can wonder ever after why the wife or husband, or whoever it might be, has not done so before. Either way, a secret which is often no longer a secret has to be regarded as one by both parties. This is, for people who love each other, as cruel a position to be in as it is possible to imagine. A cancer physician has said that relatives cannot keep a secret. 'One of the major giveaways is that people stop arguing. Things which previously always caused a family fight are now completely ignored.'[35] The doctor of the body has become a torturer of the mind.

Untold suffering must have been inflicted by this simple malpractice on the part of doctors. They have sowed distrust instead of trust. They have broken the rule of confidentiality which is one of the main principles of any medical code of ethics: they have reversed 'the usual convention of the doctor keeping confidential the information concerning an adult and telling other people only if the patient agrees'.[35] It is almost as if people who are soon to die are already dead – nurses may, for instance, take longer to answer a patient's bell call, the closer the person is to death – and the feelings of the dying do not have to be considered. Working-class people have suffered most because doctors have customarily thought of them as more 'simple', or that, with them, they can get away with it without their lack of compassion being challenged.

The rule should be not to say any more to relatives than to patients. Judging from our informants' experience, it is also far best to see patients and relatives together unless patients do not want that. When seen together, neither patient nor relatives can harbour the suspicion that the other knows more, and is withholding what they know, nor can there be a conspiracy between the family and doctors to deceive the patient into thinking they are getting better. 'As one patient sardonically remarked "I'm relieved to hear that I'm not dying of anything serious".'[36]

Ivy and Donald shared almost everything except the vital information which had stunned Ivy in the corridor. In fact, Donald knew what Ivy would not tell him and Ivy at least half-knew that Donald knew; but, although Donald gave her the chance a couple of times by broaching the subject himself, she was unable to break silence with him. She could only do this with an outsider. Commenting on the strain of not being able to talk openly, she said to the interviewer.

> It's very hard, very trying. I can't lie, I shall be glad when it's over. It's been years and I'm worn out with it.

Their situation was not made any better by the failure of their own GP to put in any appearance at home.

> My own GP, Dr S., hasn't come for two years. It's a group practice. Dr T. who gave me the letter to go into hospital is only there on Thursday evenings. He just happened to be the one when we went in. The hospital has great difficulty contacting him. Dr S. has been very nice sending round the prescriptions. The receptionist tells Dr S.; she arranges for someone to bring them round.   (Donald)

> Dr S. prescribes morphine for him but she's never been to see

him. I feel she ought to have looked in, or just rung to see how
things are.   (Ivy)

Telling all

No relative or friend should be told unless the patient is: that is
one of the cardinal rules. Another is that doctors who would
have once kept their counsel to themselves should not lean right
over the other way and tell all. It can be brutal to do so. 'It is a
chilling, cruel experience to be told of having an incurable disease
and then to be apparently dismissed with no mention of further
care, just discarded.'[38] It was rather like that with Jennifer Barnes.
Her situation was not made any better by her being a nurse and
a very experienced one at that. The doctors may have thought
that she must know what was wrong with her. But she did not.
After much toing and froing with her GP came the fateful day
when the results of a batch of tests were all to hand and she saw
her consultant to hear what they showed. All he said was that
she had 'a bit of a no-no'. Further than that was a no-go. But
how far was that? What was a no-no? Food for the imagination,
certainly. 'No-no' became a dreadful word to her which she
repeated frequently thereafter, in wonder, in anger and in scorn.
    On the following day the registrar, second only to the consult-
ant in the hierarchy, arrived at her bed and, being of an opposite
persuasion, blurted out at once the full story – cancer of the
pancreas and a secondary in the liver. 'I went completely blank
and just said yes to everything . . . . It was the end there and then
to my life.' Her son, Lee, who was visiting at the time and heard
the sentence, could not believe it and asked the registrar in his
mother's presence how long she had – the question everyone
wants to ask and few dare to. Jennifer thought, 'Please don't
answer that, I don't want to know.' She could not stop him.
The answer came, 'Maybe a couple of weeks, months, years. Some
people live a long time.' But she did not think she would. She
was too shocked to ask any questions. Later on, when she was
home again, she made an effort to understand more and asked
her GP to check for her. He phoned the consultant at the hospital
and then, instead of coming to see her, also shielded himself from
her distress by speaking to her as well over the telephone. She
broke down and couldn't take in what he said after the first few
sentences. She went completely numb. So, it seemed, did her

husband and son. The poor communication between her and the doctors created a barrier between her and her family as well.

. The doctors of Alice Colyer were more like the registrar than the consultant. She was told straight out that the growth was malignant and that she should have it out as soon as possible. Then on the day of the operation, after she had been 'starved of food and had her bowels washed out' and she was all prepared for the theatre, she got a message from the doctor (who did not come himself to give it) to say they were not going to do it after all because the cancer had spread further, to her lungs. The doctor had not looked at the x-rays done a fortnight before until just before the operation. Mrs Colyer was so affronted that the next day she got out of bed, dressed herself and walked out, never to let that doctor set his eyes on her again or she to darken the doors of that hospital again.

How terminal is terminal?

The third failing is being too precise. We have seen that Jennifer did not want to know and it was the same with Kenneth Chandler. The brother to whom he had been closest and who had also died of cancer had been given a definite term and Kenneth thought it had been awful – a sentence of death and a date for the execution. This helped to make him determined not to be the same. Whatever else was said about his prospects, he was adamant that a date should not be put on him. He mobilised his family. One of his family team of daughters talked to his doctor for him. 'On no account,' she said, 'put a time on my father.' Others, like Dermot Donoghue and Janet Rahman, both asked 'how long have I got?' almost as if life was in the doctor's gift, and perhaps even then they both wanted to know that it was not up to the doctor and to be reassured that no-one still on this earth knew the answer to their question.

Yet people feared that, without telling them, the doctors had put a time on them – that they knew more than they would say, and more accurately – and this suspicion was all the more likely to be nourished if the doctors were not generally open about the illness and its course. When they were not, ample room could be left for fantasy. One reaction was reading a special significance into what was not said. Derek Wood was worried his doctor had not forbidden him to smoke. Warnings about smoking were the stock in trade of doctors. Why had his doctor not done so? The smoke-signal must be because he was beyond saving. It must be the doctor's way of telling him. And so it went on, and on, and on, with other people.

Nothing will stop people making their own forecasts or from doing their best to falsify them. But doctors do not need to give body to them, and in any case they should not because they do not know themselves. They may be almost certain that a person has cancer, but they do not know for any particular person (as distinct from a collection of people for whom statistical probabilities can be estimated with some confidence) how long he or she has left.[39] This is partly because they do not know whether there will be a remission or not. There may even be a complete cure for an apparently incurable disorder – a miracle, as they say. It means they cannot (as long as they are truthful) kill off hope unless they are not only liars but cruel as well. It is the first duty of every doctor and every nurse not to douse hope. The most truthful and also the kindest answer to any person asking about the time put on him is 'I do not know, and cannot know.'

Making patients wait

We only mention these three failings, which coexist with the greater openness we mentioned earlier, and illustrate them from the experience of our people, because we are sure that our people are not alone. Many others have suffered, and are suffering, in the same way. What it all points to is the need for more all-round sensitivity. If that is there, all else will follow. Many doctors were exhibiting it already, at least at the level of expectations which are now common, and our people appreciated it. Other doctors do not come out so well.

Sensitivity is obviously not only wanted at the beginning of the medical relationship, although that is what we have been concentrating on. The diagnosis, as we saw in the last chapter, marks the start of what can be a protracted, though intermittent, interaction. Patients need information, and to be able to get information at almost any point, about new symptoms, treatments, side effects, income maintenance, and about any help they can get from outside in making adaptations in their lives. It always matters how the information is given. Openness can be undone or even wounding if doctors deliver themselves from on high, as if in public, especially if in fact in public. However truthful such doctors are, their patients may then be struck deaf. They are more likely to take it in if the relationship is a bit more like that between ordinary people, with more informality to it, so that the doctors can be regarded, without being over-familiar, more as people than as awesome authorities; for that to happen the doctors need to treat their patients more as persons too than as vexing claimants on their time. The balance of power needs to be changed, and this requires the right training and the right attitude.

It calls for much more effort to be put into finding out how some very busy doctors still manage to give the impression to their patients that there is no rush. It is partly a matter of concentration, of putting everything out of mind except the patient before them. As Cicely Saunders said, 'Time isn't a question of length. It's a question of depth, isn't it? It's how completely you listen that counts.'[40] But there is more to it than just concentration. Research is needed so that good practice can become more systematic. As things are now, the time that a patient has with a consultant at a hospital is often so brief as to rule out openness of a sensitive kind. Doctors should have time not only to listen but to give patients the chance to ask questions – in other words not be hurried, or give the impression of being hurried – and make a special effort, backed up by decent telephone or other interpreting services, when the patient is from an ethnic minority and does not speak English.[41] They should, ideally, also have time to talk to carers. Doctors, although with all the power over treatment, are five-minutes-a-month people whereas the carers may be 24-hours-a-day people and therefore know a great deal about the patient's condition, but need to be a friend too.

Getting to the hospital

In all spheres of life important people demonstrate their status according to the common time-measure.[42] They show in a hundred ways how valuable their time is compared to that of those with whom they have to deal, by being unavailable except by appointment, by making people wait for the appointment (partly because scarce resources arc rationed by making people wait) and by giving no more than a minimal amount of time to those they admit to their presence. What all high-status people do, hospital doctors in the Health Service do in excelsis. There is therefore a chronic imbalance between the value put on patients' time – tending to zero – and the value put on doctors' time – tending to infinity.

The negligible value of their time is brought forcefully home to patients well before they get to the hospital. Journeys short in miles can be inordinately long in time, especially for people without the use of a car or the ability to bend sufficiently to get into them. After days or weeks of fearful anticipation of the day of the oracle, the dread of it is not lessened by having to wait, and wait. Ambulances which collect people for out-patient appointments are not 999 ambulances. They are buses without timetables and without regular routes. They pick up one person after another from wherever they may be before driving with their load to the hospital. Since every day's round is different, the time, even the approximate time, of their call may not be known in advance. The patient has to be dressed and waiting by the door from the earliest hour that the ambulance might come for fear that if they are not, the ambulancemen, also pressed for time, will knock and then without waiting for the patient to shuffle up the passage drive off without them. If that happens, the patient may have to wait weeks, even months, for another appointment and the treatment be dangerously delayed. Imagine the stress for a tired and ill person on their own in the winter and knowing they have not long to live, sitting hour by hour in a cold hallway by the door desperately trying not to nod off.

The last occasion Arthur Jacobs had been for his check-up it was much as usual. 'When I went to the hospital last Friday I was ready at 8.30 a.m. for the ambulance and it arrived at 11.30. Then when I'd finished I waited to come home for two hours.' Donald Knight's ambulance called at eight in the morning and he did not get back till eight at night for a journey of four or five miles. For the return journey people could only hope they would be able to move when the ambulance was ready and not be struggling with the violent diarrhoea that sometimes followed a chemo-therapy treatment. Janet Rahman had an attack while she was waiting and feared she would miss the ambulance altogether. Others were afraid they would soil their clothes and upset other patients travelling with them.

It could be still worse if there weren't any ambulances. There was none for Dermot the first time he left hospital. He was discharged with hardly any notice, after four or five weeks in which he had had a drastic operation to get at a cancer lying at the back of his stomach, and only two days after a battery of tubes to different parts of his body had been disconnected. He had eaten hardly anything for weeks and yet he was discharged at a few hours' notice. The hospital gave him a stick and sent him out on a cold winter's day to walk home. Every step tugged at his stitches and his wound. He had diarrhoea on the way. When he reached home no-one was there – he lived alone – and there was no food. In his exhausted state all he could do was drop on to his bed and wait and wonder whether there was any point even in hope. Fortunately, on the next day the lady from the landing above did look in to see if he was back and fetched him some food. If it had not been for her, or other neighbours, he could have died of starvation instead of cancer.

Multiple doctors

Patients have to wait, for an appointment to be given, to get to the hospital, and to be seen when there, and after all that, *your* doctor may have no time for you. He or she is simply not there, and in his or her place is another doctor you have never seen before. The experience can be exasperating. It was for Julia Searle. 'I knew it was going to be an important consultation because I knew they had the results of all the tests and I knew that the treatment would have to be decided. I found myself with a completely new doctor. It's most disturbing to see a different doctor every time you go.' Likewise for Carol Taylor. 'When you have a different doctor walk in it throws you off key.' With her usual consultant, 'I can recall with him and I'm confident he knows everything about me.' Her memory was supported by being shared with another memory which tallied with her own. When a new doctor was flicking through the notes and asking her questions that she'd answered many times before 'whatever you were going to say goes completely from your mind'. If the doctor does not even have the notes and the patient has to go over her medical history once again it can be too much. But for Carol there was also a rather perverse gain in seeing different doctors who said slightly different things. It helped her to remain in a state of confusion and make out that the outlook was bright when it wasn't. She was also able to play off one doctor against another.

On one of Kenneth Chandler's many visits to hospital he saw a new doctor who didn't even have on the table the enormous wodge of notes which normally sat there. They had been lost, temporarily. The new doctor apparently thought that Kenneth needed a kidney test.

> He said a kidney test, and I said, what for? I'm not complaining about my kidneys. How can he ask me to have something done and he doesn't know my full history?

It was only later that he discovered it was normal to have a kidney condition for someone in his state. It happened again to him with yet another new doctor.

> It was a complete and utter waste of time. It was a new doctor and I might just as well have talked to these flowers (indicating some chrysanthemums). It's very frustrating – not that I wanted to be prodded about. I think his mind was on other things.

It was even worse for Janet Rahman. Her ordinary consultant had not told her to have chemotherapy. But on one of her hospital visits he was not there. She saw another doctor and he referred her for chemo. Was she to accept it? The chemo, with all its side effects, was started but, after a few treatments, she stopped it herself. It was not clear what her 'own' consultant would have wanted. But her confidence in him, and his judgement, had been undermined.

The asymmetry of time

The way the system works, the one message which is drummed into people is that doctors, and above all the consultants at the top of the hierarchy, have very little or even no time for them while they, on the other hand, though with little time left, are expected to put all theirs at the disposal of the system. The imbalance is extreme, so much so that when some of the patients finally arrived in the consulting room, especially when they came alone, they were shaking with fatigue and too exhausted to absorb any information whatsoever or to give it, including information about new symptoms which could be crucial for the decisions taken by the doctor.[43] They sometimes had to wait for further hours in the out-patient department after arriving in the hospital and having several tests done – a blood count, an x-ray – before they got their three minutes with the doctor.

The routine would be tiring for a young and healthy person; how much more so for someone desperately ill, frightened and made to feel of no account by the extraordinary contrast between the value of the doctor's time and their own. For the doctor, the patient could be just one in a stream of dozens of anxious people seen on one crowded day; for the patient, it could be the most important event in a month, or even in a lifetime.

But, despite the imbalance, unless they were not told anything of significance to them or treated discourteously, the patients with so much time were not critical of the consultants with so little. They needed the doctor more than the doctor needed them. They had got used to the short time he had – it was nearly always a he. They sometimes adjusted by not taking up his time with a report of their symptoms. But they were critical of the general arrangements which took up so much of their day that they were exhausted. It could take four days or more to recover from a four-minute appointment, although there could also be an immediate relief in leaving the consultant's room at all without being whipped deeper into the recesses of the hospital from which there might be no return.

All this is not news to the consultants. Most of them know that the rush is unsatisfactory and only put up with it because they have to. If they give more time to one person they will keep another person waiting longer and get behind with everyone. Many consultants have private patients as well and know that, if they could treat their NHS patients as though private and give them as much time, it would be better – although worse for their earnings from their private practice. Private patients can be worse off in many ways – other specialists are not as available as they would be in a hospital; they are in their private rooms not so much noticed by the nurses; they do not have the benefit of belonging to an informal group of patients, a camaraderie, which acts as an advisory forum. But they do see the same doctor at each appointment; they can get early appointments at times that suit themselves; they do not have to sit waiting for so long, and their consultants will make appointments for them with other doctors.[44] Above all, they have more time with him. The consultants know that at least would be better. They may also know that, for their NHS patients as much as for any other, the key to good communication is not so much talking as listening, and always asking the patients if they have any questions or (at the end of the appointment) any *further* questions to ask. But they may have no time to listen. There are just too many patients.

The NHS is always short of resources, which means above all a shortage of doctors and nurses whose wages make up a good part of the whole cost. The chronic shortage of money creates the chronic imbalance between the time-availability of the two parties, at least as the system is organised at present. The resources have to be rationed and if it is not done by money, as it would be if people had to pay for their own medical care, it has to be done by forcing people to wait. If waiting lists are long before admission, some people will have got better or died or moved before their turn comes. If people have to wait for hours in out-patients, it means that the doctors can be continuously at work. There is no danger of *them* having to wait.

But there is still the question of whether, even within the limits set by present resources, communication could be improved by deploying the resources differently. It is obviously right that the most important decisions about treatment should be taken by consultants: they are the most experienced doctors. But it does not follow that they should be the only people to pass on information. For this there can, and should, be delegation to junior doctors and, above all, to nurses. Their great advantage is that, pressed though they are too, they are around when the ward is less busy and when visitors are there.

But delegation cannot work well unless it is part of a more comprehensive policy for communication within a hospital department, ideally including GPs as well.[45] As long as the rule is that all key information should come from the consultant there does not have to be a plan: that *is* the plan, but one with a great weakness, especially if other staff do not know what the consultant has said.

> The doctors say things to the patient and the relatives and then they leave the ward. Then you are left with the relatives and you feel very limited because you don't know what the doctor has said. You have to tread very carefully, because you

don't know what in the relative's mind is based upon fact and what is based upon fantasy.[46]

Once there is a policy, and that must cover delegation, it has to be decided which other members of the staff shall be responsible for giving what information, and how best to give them the training they will need. To do this is not all that formidable. At St Christopher's Hospice, everything that has been said to a patient about his illness is written down on an information sheet, and any member of the staff looks at it before speaking to the patient. Working for the College of Health, Michael Young prepared a scheme for a hospital which did provide for delegation.[47] On their discharge from hospital patients had an interview which was not necessarily with the consultant. They were told

• why they had been admitted to hospital
• what was found and done to them
• what they and their family could do to help their recovery at home.

Patients, as well as being told, received a written record of what was said, and could, if they wished, have the conversation recorded and put on a tape which they could take home with them. The tapes were found particularly valuable by relatives.[48] In the Grantham study mentioned above 'A majority of those who listened to their tape said that someone else had also heard it. Most commonly this was their spouse, but other family members, friends, work colleagues and neighbours had also heard tapes.'

However much is said, written records are needed as well. The NHS *Guide to Consent*, which was quoted earlier in the chapter, went on to say that 'Oral or written consent should be recorded in the patient's notes with relevant details of the health professional's explanation.'[49] It is only a step from there to recording all the vital information which is given. If that were done, then the patient could have the record and any doctor or nurse as well. It is a sign of the times, and of the greater general openness, that the Access to Health Records Act of 1990 gave individuals the right of access to their health records. The patient now has a right to see them and have them photocopied. As yet few patients know about this. Doctors seldom tell them. But if they get to know, and become used to having and carrying their own records, and get more experience in understanding them, it could in itself make a substantial difference. For one thing it would not matter so much if, as frequently happens, their notes are lost in the hospital, nor if a patient is seen by a stand-in doctor and that doctor knows little or nothing about what has happened before. We say this knowing that by and large doctors have been reluctant to abandon paper for electronics. But when they do, and use the power of computers to the full and give patients access to them, the patients should be on the way to having at hand not just one paper record at a particular time but a continuous record of their relationship with the NHS in its many different departments and activities. For that to happen the patients will need training too.

* * *

The relationship is unequal between laypeople and the experts who know so much more about our bodies than we know ourselves. People on the fast track to death have been deprived of some of the power they had, or seemed to have, when they were still on the standard slower route which constitutes health. They are relatively powerless, and feel it, and feel it more if doctors and others are not open with them.

The reassurances they need were once given by another kind of expert. Priests were the experts in death. Being holy men, they were credited with having some privileged access to the mysteries, and something of what they understood could be passed on to anyone who had the same kind of faith they had themselves. After their fashion they were taken to understand, even sometimes to mediate, death. But most of the new experts, who know with so much more precision about dying, do not claim to understand anything about death. Their hard-won expertise is in how to stave it off. They are the anti-death experts. But they have at least one of the vital attributes of the holy men who knew about death. They still retain some of the aura of the miracle worker.[50] But the new openness which has ousted much of the magic has the great advantage that, once the authority given by silence has gone, there can be open discussion. The open discussion will give rise to new questions, and, perhaps, new answers. The new openness means that the nature of what is considered a good death is still changing, fast.

Chapter 6

Pain and euthanasia

We have described how the patients, and their carers, and their doctors, managed so far, without more than mentioning pain. Pain from cancer can be much better controlled than it used to be. But it has not been eliminated; nor have other kinds of pain caused by surgery and other treatments. Nor, surprisingly, do people (at any rate the people in our study) want it to be eliminated.

The future was another matter. Almost everyone had something to say about the time when they would be nearer death. For instance, about their fear:

> I hate pain. I'm not sure I have a fear of dying. It's the manner and the possibility of a lot of pain.   (Janet)

Harold said much the same thing, about not wanting to suffer much and for long. 'I'm not afraid of dying, it's the method of dying. The only thing that worries me is that I don't want to last too long when the pain is too bad.' Neither Harold nor anyone else had read what has been said on the subject by one of the outstanding experts on the matter: that cancer patients at any rate can be 'reassured that the moment of death from cancer is almost invariably peaceful'.[1]

The fear did not come from anything experienced up to that point so much as from an expectation of what they might yet have coming to them. They were frightened that when they got worse the pain would too, and would, eventually, get out of control. But for the moment they could fend off that fear and show they were not that far gone by controlling their pain. It was an expression of their independence. They had the means of asserting and reassuring themselves. This they could most readily do when the pain was induced by something they themselves did, for example, by getting out of bed in the morning. This was a bad time of the day for almost everyone, causing (as we said in Chapter 3) all manner of little or not so little discomforts.

> I'm afraid to wake up because I think 'oh, please don't start'. It takes a lot out of you.   (Kenneth)

But if they took it all gently, and took frequent rests, they would usually be able to manage, and without the discomfort. If not they could take a little medication.

They could do the same when they over-extended themselves in the day, by eating for the sake of conviviality a bigger lunch than they really wanted, by the sort of shopping expedition that still meant so much to Julia, or by struggling to take a walk to show themselves they still had some strength left. If they came back in pain, a small dose of pain-killer could bring it under control. As Harold said,

> I usually take my medication after I've been out. The walk is painful but I put up with that. I don't want to dose up. That's the slippery slope.

The weekend could also be the same kind of ordeal, willingly endured, indeed eagerly looked forward to. Relatives would come. Children would play and make a noise. It was delightful as well as tiring; but afterwards there could be a reaction and the pain could flare up again. Harold:

> Sunday was bad but it was a reaction to Saturday. You get tense and that causes trouble. If I can, I like to put up with a certain amount of pain and then I think I must take the pain-killers straight away.

The regular pain with a known cause and largely within their control was much easier to deal with than the sort they were liable to have in hospital. An operation was an unknown, a little death, and no-one could know for sure what was on the other side, when they hoped to wake up from the sleep into which they had been plunged by a higher power. We have already described Dermot's fear of another torment after his third operation, and others were the same. It was partly the uncertainty of it – waiting to hear if the operation had been 'successful' or had revealed, when internal organs were bared to sight, some new complication hidden from the search by x-rays, scanners and ultrasounds. It was partly the pain that could follow it which might be too much for the hospital doctors and far too much for the patient. The control, if any, would then be in someone else's hands. Julia was very sorry she could not have another operation when at last no more could be done for her. But at least she would not have to face that kind of pain again.

> The fear I had of pain has gone now. I don't wake in the morning and my stomach sinks because I have to have the operation.

There was, however, still the middle of the night when people were alone and could not distract themselves.

> If you're in a lot of pain but keep chatting you can often get through it whereas if you're alone with no distraction the pain becomes all important.   (Julia)

Levels of pain

The same issue of control kept coming up about the levels of pain. It was common to take smaller doses of pain-killers than the doctors had prescribed. Once they had assured themselves that pain was controllable – could be reduced if it got worse – they chose to tolerate it.

> When it gets to a certain pitch I fall back on it. There are times when it is more than I can stomach and I look for relief but I don't run for the bottle every time I get some pain. (Kenneth)

At one stage Kenneth not only avoided running for the bottle, he took himself off the morphine completely. The Home Care nurse asked him why. He said he didn't think he needed it, and, he might have said, he could hope that he was improving. Drug intake was a measuring rod. Taking less was progress, more decline. It was as if the pain belonged to death, and if it could be managed without artificial aid, or with less, it meant that death was not so near. If this is the attitude, then the message from the hospice at St Christopher's – that cancer pain can be cut right down by opiates – is not going to penetrate all that quickly, as perhaps it should not if it reduces the measure of control that people have.

All this could be exasperating for the carer. Jackie said of her mother:

> I encouraged her to take her pain medication continually but she took it spasmodically. She thought that if she could withstand it then she was getting better. She felt good about it when she managed without it.

But it was, if anything, comforting for the patients, especially if they could achieve the same result by other means.

> I didn't take my top up dose. Instead, I tried some self-help and relaxation. I kept telling myself, 'Let it wash over you, leave it', and I actually fell asleep and woke up and the pain had gone. I was very pleased.   (Julia)

Knowing that the pain could be damped down was what mattered. People were continually seeking virtuous spirals in which reduced pain reduced anxiety, and reduced anxiety reduced pain.[2] The pain-killers could often have their effect less by being used than by being available. Moreover, patients were not inclined to believe doctors who said the drugs were not addictive. They thought they were, and that less of them now meant they would be building up a sort of investment for the future – which they could draw on when they really needed the drugs most and they would still be effective.

Not, of course, that it always worked: when it didn't a vicious instead of a virtuous spiral could be set in motion. The same Julia on another occasion told us:

> I'm burnt out with pain. The whole year has been full of a lot of bad pain. It was partly my fault because I wouldn't take the dose I needed to get rid of it so I'm increasingly frightened about pain now and I can't cope as well as I did. Even the idea of taking off the bandages on my arm fills me with apprehension. It's going to hurt and I'm not going to like it. I've just had enough.

Physical pain and state of mind were inseparable from each other.[3]

All in all, people seemed to manage it well, partly, perhaps, because, in the light of the fearsome reputation of cancer, they

expected the pain would be so much worse. But they were reckoning without the new treatments which have been produced;
they belong fair and square to the new branch of medicine,
palliative medicine.[4] Its pioneers have declared that cancer pain
can now be largely brought under control. What Saunders and
her colleagues have shown is that it is easier to keep people free
from pain by regular small doses of morphine before the pain
builds up, and that morphine given for pain is less likely to
produce addiction than morphine given for other reasons. In the
minority who need larger and larger doses the body's increasing
tolerance of the drug often enables pain relief to be secured
without suffering any particular confusion. If the people in our
study are a good guide, much pain has been relieved in the best
way possible, not only by the direct pharmacological effect of the
drugs but also by the effect of pharmacology on psychology.
The drugs being available, people have been able to extend their
control over something which is in any case highly personal and
idiosyncratic. No doctor knows how much pain you have; only
you know that, and if you can vary the level, and explore it, you
can exercise some autonomy in a matter that is quite vital to
you. The pain is almost welcome because you have the freedom
to feel pain, or not, as you wish.

'How will I know I'm in pain if I continually take a pain-
killer?' asked Carol. They were not just tolerating pain, their
experience was more positive than that.

> You need pain so you are aware you are alive. Everyone says,
> 'do you have any pain?' anxiously. It should be the other way
> round.   (Julia)

So far this summary of what our people said about pain suggests
one particular condition of a good death – not that it should be
without pain but that, as far as possible, the pain should be under
the control of the patient and that the patient should be to some
degree in control at the moment of death. To be in that position
is another assertion of the underlying wish for independence.

Euthanasia

But if the extent of pain should be for the patient to decide,
should not also the decision whether to end the pain, or multiple
distress, by ending the carrier of the pain? There is only one sure

way of bringing an end to the distress associated with death. Hence the relevance of the ongoing debate about euthanasia. Literally, from its Greek origin (in the same family of words as eulogy or eucharist or euphonious), the word means a good or easy death, and in that sense euthanasia is the subject of the whole book and many others besides. But it has taken on a more restricted meaning: voluntary and assisted euthanasia. The connection has been made in a particular manner by Cicely Saunders. She argues that because the right regime can now overcome pain and much of the distress that would otherwise have gone with it, there is no need for euthanasia;[5] and the hospice movement, as one of the contemporary reforming movements to do with death, has been set in opposition to euthanasia as another reforming movement. Dr Twycross asserted, in similar vein, that there is now no need for euthanasia but for educating the medical profession and improving services in general so that the practice of a place like St Christopher's Hospice can be made available to all.[6] A hospice could be considered a place for euthanasia in its original Greek sense.

If it had not been for the experience of one of our informants, we might have left it at that and not felt any need to venture into this arena at all. But the Allens bid us otherwise. We know they are not alone. A large-scale survey has been made in which relatives and others close to people who had died were asked about that person's wishes and their own. 'About a quarter of both respondents and the people who died expressed the view that an earlier death would be, or would have been, preferable.'[7] This does not mean that they would have welcomed euthanasia, but it is a sizeable expression of dissatisfaction with the time taken to die.

Harold demonstrated that, despite what hospice people say, there is more to consider than pain, at any rate what is called physical pain. He was unusual in wanting to die, and wanting help in doing so, but except in degree not in the distress he experienced. Breathlessness was common amongst the patients, and even the threat of it was distressing.

> I am afraid of having an attack of breathlessness. It can happen at any time. I have an immediate response. I immediately take out my teeth when it happens.   (Derek)

Swelling of the feet and limbs was equally common.

My right arm has been up and down. I can't put it out straight you see. It's the weight that's the trouble. It's like a heavy bag of potatoes.   (Janet)

Then there was the sickness.

The constant nausea and sickness is very debilitating. Pain is easier to cope with.   (Julia)

There is also the distress caused by the loss of faculties. In the later stages of his illness – we have touched on this already – Harold underwent an acceleration in his decline. He could not see, hear, move or concentrate for more than a short time. Life became too much for him to want to cling to it. The crucial thing was that he knew he was becoming more of a burden to his wife and family. He did not want to be. He wanted it over with, and said so forthrightly to the Home Care nurse who was visiting him regularly. She parried lightly, saying we all have to go sometime. This upset him even more. He thought that for the first time in his dealings with her she lacked understanding of what it was like for *him*. He got very cross.

He talked about it with Lilian. She was convinced and they asked their superb GP if he could help Harold to escape from his distress. He could not. 'We can't ask him what he can't do. He's explained that his task is to make me as painfree and as comfortable as possible.'   Harold and Lilian accepted this – not just because they had to, for they respected their doctor and his position, and understood it – but without altering their views. Harold said several times he wished he was dead. They had both belonged to a church but the experience of those final weeks robbed Harold of his faith, and nearly did the same for Lilian. Harold stopped taking Communion. Lilian: 'I just want it finished. I don't like seeing him suffer like this.'

After Harold died, Lilian had no regrets at all about the last year as a whole – the year of his miraculous reprieve – but she did, and many, about his last few weeks.

I still definitely think that they ought to make it easy. It's not right at all. When patients get to that stage you know jolly well that it is only a matter of hours or days and it's going to happen anyway. I love animals and I don't like to see them suffer but at least you can put them out of their misery. Some people say, 'oh, it's terrible to even think of it' but I think if

those people watched someone in that situation I think they
might think twice. It's certainly changed my way of thinking.
I know he (doctor) felt awful about not being able to do
anything.

I think it was because, in spite of all the medical care and
doing the utmost to relieve suffering, it was horrific still. That's
what I found hard to accept – that that could be allowed to
happen.

If the patients themselves wish it, I don't think we should
begrudge anybody to have a dignified exit from life, and no
way do they die with dignity and no-one can make me believe
otherwise. The trouble is, until you experience it, you don't
believe it.

Had he died sooner, Lilian's bereavement might have been a
little easier. We will come back to this in the next chapter. She
felt guilty for having let it happen and for not having the courage
to take the action she wanted to, like the young people she read
about in the newspaper who had helped their mother to die.

Legalised?

People can sometimes bring on a death by surrendering the will
to live. If they could always do so, euthanasia would not be an
issue. We would not have expected that amongst the fourteen
patients there would be many who wanted euthanasia. They were,
on the whole, being well looked after. Harold, despite the care
he was receiving, was very much the exception. The Allen family
therefore raise once again the thorny set of questions which have
become more and more widely discussed. Should euthanasia, with
all the necessary safeguards, be legalised? Perhaps on the model
of what has happened in Holland? There, the Dutch courts have
allowed euthanasia where there is 'a concrete expectation of
death', if there is 'unbearable suffering', 'psychic suffering' and
'potential disfigurement of personality'.[8] These all involve
decisions which can only be based on the subjective judgements
of doctors; but Harold would surely have qualified if he had been
Dutch. The Dutch experience does not, however, all point one
way. It is said that euthanasia outside the law has also become
more readily tolerated. It is notable that Holland has fewer hospices and palliative care units than any other country in Europe.

The arguments, for and against, have been gone over many times before, for instance by the Institute of Medical Ethics,[9] speaking for the pros, and the BMA[10] and a Select Committee on Medical Ethics of the House of Lords[11] speaking for those against. The statement of the problem, if not the conclusion, in the first report would be accepted by many.

> The lives of an increasing number of patients, predominantly but by no means all elderly, are now being prolonged by modern medicine in states of coma, severe incapacity, or pain they consider unrelievable and from which they seek release. Doctors in charge of such patients have to decide not only whether they are morally bound to continue with life-prolonging treatment, but also, if no such treatment is being given, whether and in what circumstances it is ethical to hasten their deaths by administration of narcotic drugs.

In a debate following the House of Lords report, Lord Alport said that people used to look forward to death because life was nasty, brutish and short.[12] Now 'Owing to the advances in medical technology, life for an increasing number of people is nasty, brutish and long.'

There are a wide range of reactions to the problem. There is the simple and persuasive case for liberty. Why should Harold or anyone else be prevented from exercising what should be a fundamental liberty, to die? We do not have freedom of choice about whether to come into existence at the beginning of life, nor from whose womb to make our impressive entrance; but at the other end of life should we not be free to go out of existence at least of an earthly sort, if it has become too difficult to bear? The very achievements of medicine help to strengthen the argument. A stock nightmare of modern times is of doctors in possession of the power to keep us alive when our bodies are at least partly dead, trussed up with tubes to put in and draw out fluids and to keep the semblance of life going with the aid of life-support machines of frightening ingenuity. The prospect of being kept alive against one's will (or when one is not in any position to express it) is more frightening than the prospect of being killed.

The power put at the disposal of a doctor by modern science and technology has given a new twist to the old relationship between liberty and the sanctity of life. Medicine has advanced, even in a century when there have also been so many barbaric killings, because the sanctity of life has been at the root of the worldwide covenant between doctor and patient, in evidence even on the battlefield. We put ourselves in the hands of doctors because we have faith, if not necessarily in their skill then certainly in their benevolent intentions and in the belief that their intentions coincide with our hopes. We hope to live: they help us to do so, and so we go to them reasonably confident that they will do their best for us. Whatever the moral breakdown in other spheres, the concordance between the parties to the two sides of the relationship – the generality of patients and possible patients and the specialists of medicine – has given it great prominence in the general hierarchy of values. Without this agreement modern societies would be a good deal more fragile than they are. The unwritten compact, with elements of the sacred to it, has made health care one of the world's biggest industries, driven continuously by its internal dynamic to add to its ever-expanding empire.

But its success is no triumph. The basic assumption underlying the compact can no longer be taken for granted. It is not only the fear of the life-support machine. All the other tools and skills of modern medicine have kept more and more people alive but without necessarily restoring them to a full life. More patients are caught up in lingering illnesses and disabilities.[13] In these circumstances a life does not always appear so sacred; it may have lost its quality. Death can then in a way seem more sacred than life, or at any rate a blessed way of putting someone out of their misery. So it is partly the advance of medicine, motivated by the respect for life, which has raised the age-old issue of suicide in a new form. Should people have, or as far as earthly powers allow be deprived of, the liberty to die if they have reversed the usual preference and consider life the threat and death the mercy?

The freedom to die can be presented as a proper extension of all that was said in Chapter 5 about the new kind of relationship in which patients are taken into the confidence of doctors and told as much as they can take in about their illness. If it is accepted that there should be no 'invasion' of their bodies without their explicit consent, patients must understand enough to be able to give this consent knowingly. Under this regime they are 'offered' operations, not told they are to have them. But if doctors continue to develop a laudable frankness until near the end, even though they must never say outright there is no hope, they are sometimes bound, if only by a look or a change in the tone of voice, to indicate that the best they can do is to soften the death that is to come. If the patient then turns to the doctor and says – 'in that case I don't want to live, and I need you to help me as you have done your best to help me up to this point' – is the doctor also bound to reply, like Harold's doctor, that this is a kind of medical help he is forbidden to, and cannot, give? Is the doctor to be unable to do what he or she sometimes must know is in the patient's best interest, which up to this moment has been the lodestar?

The plea for this mortal liberty is all the more telling because it cannot easily be argued that it would be used wantonly, as if self-preservation were not the ground-work of our lives until faced with such a predicament. People may make mistakes, of course, for instance by believing, when they are deeply depressed, that they will not be able to emerge from it except through suicide – this when the means of alleviating depression are to hand even for terminal patients.[14] But at any rate some of those who want to commit suicide are not clinically depressed and do not make their exit for frivolous reasons. It is not just that they want to get rid of the pain which the hospices, and their domiciliary assistants, can to some extent control. They have been bent lower and lower by an accumulation of distress which can be far more formidable in its totality than the sort of pain which opiates can relieve and, above all, they can fear becoming more and more dependent on their carers, losing all their independence and eventually becoming too much of a burden to bear.[15] The plea for liberty is a cry for help. If the function of doctors is to help their patients, how can they justify making no response?

It can, indeed, be claimed that, as with many other rules which were once the unquestioned imperatives of a traditional order, to ask the question is also to answer it. Suicide was regarded as a sin of the most grievous kind as long as the rationale for doing so did not have to be spelt out. Moral truths are at their most impregnable when they do not have to be buttressed by reason. But as the religious underpinning for the prohibition has been relaxed and doctors' undemocratic right to silence began to be questioned, the old doctrine could be less and less taken for granted. The doctrine has been losing its shield of infallibility, and, once open to attack, has had to give ground, inch by painful inch.

The delicate balance

Despite the undoubted force in an individualistic society of the libertarian case for absolute power over death to be added to relative power over life, the main drift of this book is against it. The case as customarily made is all to do with individuals – the individual's right to die, the individual's right to know and to decide – yet we have been pointing out, again and again, that patients are not necessarily on their own. They are often members of family and other social groups, and the interests and influence of these groups have to be considered before any rounded view can be taken about a suicide which removes from life not only an individual but a member of a group and a society.

For their own protection groups are prophylactics against suicide, and the firmer they are in the loyalty they generate, the more powerfully they act to save life. The sociologist, Émile Durkheim, pointed out that 'Suicide varies inversely with the degree of integration of the social groups of which the individual forms a part.'[16] The research on the mortality of widowers which was mentioned earlier[17] extends this proposition from suicides to all deaths, or at least does so in a particular set of circumstances by showing that the loss of close relatives generates more deaths amongst the survivors. One death gives rise to another, and it is also true that one life supports another. The persistence of life derives from the presence of group support.

In an integrated group there is a collective will to live. The loss of any one of its members is a threat to the whole, and each has an interest in preserving the lives of the others. Hence the general condemnation of suicide in almost all societies. The survivors of suicide, or of any death, can suffer much more than the dead, and so can be specially keen to avoid it. The collective will to live translates itself into an individual will to live. Bettelheim wrote about his experiences as a prisoner in Auschwitz, but what he said has some general significance.

The sheer will to live cannot take the place of the strength one derives from outside support, real or imagined. This is why those . . . who lovingly work for one's return to the living are the strongest lifeline imaginable, the most powerful motive for staying alive.[18]

The issue about euthanasia is also a collective matter because the advances in medicine have put a greater burden on carers. Lingering illnesses are bound to. The patient suffering from them has to recognise that the illness is a burden (and would be even more so if he .or she did not recognise it), and the carer likewise, although a burden that is usually borne readily enough, even with a hopeful heart. But we do not draw the conclusion that, for the sake of the carers, euthanasia should be made easier, but rather the opposite. Families would have to agree to it, and would then feel responsible, and guilty, which could make the whole bereavement (which causes more misery than terminal illness) generally more painful. They would be bound to ask themselves whether the death was the result of their lack of love. Euthanasia could make family relationships still more delicate than they are liable to be anyway. This is why, having seen so much of the carers, we fear that a general option of euthanasia, unless surrounded by the most stringent safeguards, would do more harm than good.

The peace of mind which is both so desirable and so difficult to achieve for a person so ill would be more fraught if the patients were all the time wondering whether, for the sake of their carers, they should seek an earlier death than nature unaided will grant them. The right to die could become a duty to die. It could nag continuously, so much so as to make the last phase of life a torment on that score alone. If a decision had to be made, and it went against euthanasia, the patient could be wretchedly guilty for continuing to put such a burden on those around. However loving, few carers could forbear from wondering sometimes whether an end would not be merciful. If it were easy for this to happen, carers could ponder it much more, and that could undermine the relationship with the patient, even where they loved each other. If they did not, the dangers are obvious.

In the future there are not going to be so many relatives to share the burden of care. More is going to fall on one or a few, and these few, perhaps with a less deep sense of obligation, may buckle under the strain and nudge towards euthanasia for their own sake, rather than for the sake of the patient. Some of them might even be tempted for reasons even less worthy, like greed for the property that would come to them after the death. The very old could be particularly vulnerable, as was suggested by the study we have already cited.

> The results support the view that in present-day society increasing age is associated with a greater likelihood of being seen as a burden by other family members, friends and others. The very old are less likely to have spouses who will value the continuation of their life or who will miss them a great deal when they are gone. The children of those who die, as well as other family members, friends and officials, who are perhaps less emotionally close to the dying than spouses, or whose lives are made particularly difficult by the burden of caring, are more likely to feel that it would have been better if the person had died earlier than they did.[19]

A wider acceptance of euthanasia would have the further danger that it could undermine the trust that people feel, and need to feel, in their doctors. Even as the law and practice are now, many patients already believe that doctors practise euthanasia, and are frightened they may become the victims. Some doctors are very cautious about giving injections. They have come across the notion that injections may be intended to be fatal. If there were a more liberal attitude to euthanasia, and the consequence was to increase this sort of suspicion, that would indeed be a bitter outcome. But it would not necessarily follow. The suspicion may be there partly because euthanasia has at present to be kept dark and hidden. If it were out in the open, and recognised, and stringent procedures were laid down which patients knew about, anxiety might be less, not more.

If the general prohibition against euthanasia seems right, for the peace of mind of patients and of most carers, there have to be some exceptions which deserve to be treated differently from the general run – this where the patient is suffering from great distress, even agony, mental or physical, and the carers are having to watch over what seems like pointless suffering without being able to offer any relief. It could be a collective torture that is being imposed. Ludovic Kennedy refers his readers to the plight of one of his correspondents who wrote:

> I myself went through a harrowing experience with my beloved mother's final years. To see someone you love suffering and

daily getting worse is torture. She had very bad and very painful rheumatoid arthritis for several years before finally coming to live with us. The cortisone she was prescribed effectively destroyed her body, but death seemed as far off as ever. At last she said, 'Tonight I'm going to do it, I'm going to cut my arteries in my arm.' I never felt more helpless, more grief stricken. I lay in bed in the next room while she tried to kill herself with a pair of scissors. The horror of that night thirty years ago will be with me forever. In the morning she was still alive.[20]

It would have been more merciful if euthanasia had been available for her, and for Harold.

Since no government is likely to grasp the nettle, the practical question is how the common law as declared in the courts will (and should) develop. It is axiomatic for the law as well as medical practice that patients cannot be treated at all without their consent. They can, if they have their wits about them, ask that treatment be suspended even though it means that they die. If this be suicide, it is a form of suicide that is open to anyone being kept alive only by their treatment. But if people can kill themselves in this way (passive euthanasia, as it is called) by removing themselves from their doctors, is it such a big step to lend them the assistance of doctors (positive euthanasia) to achieve the same end?

Another Kennedy, Ian, Professor of Medical Law and Ethics in King's College, London, has argued that the gap between passive and active becomes narrower as soon as it is recognised that, as the law stands, doctors are fully entitled to do all that they can do to reduce pain, even if the drugs they use bring on death.[21] He postulates two doctors.

Dr A and Dr B are in all respects similar. They are caring, respected doctors with impeccable backgrounds. Dr A's patient, Mr X, is suffering from a fatal illness which is now in its final stages. He is near to death and in great pain. He can also see the pain his suffering is causing to his family who maintain a vigil at his bedside. He asks Dr A to put him out of his misery. Dr A explains that he cannot do so, but that he will steadily increase the amount of pain relieving drugs which Mr X receives. The effect of this, Dr A explains, will be that over a period of time, perhaps a few days, the dose prescribed will be such that Mr X will in fact die, albeit, he adds, as a consequence of the attempt to relieve pain. Two days later Mr X dies. Meanwhile Dr B's patient, Mrs Z, is in virtually the same situation. In response to her entreaties Dr B says that he will give her something which will bring her the relief and release she seeks. Dr B injects Mrs Z with potassium chloride. She dies within minutes, a rapid end to her pain and suffering.

Kennedy contrasts the two cases, almost identical in their main details, except that Mr X took much longer to die and Dr A used a recognised pain-killing drug whereas Dr B did not. But the law regards Dr B as a murderer and Dr A as a perfectly reasonable doctor. The argument is that the drug used to bring on death cannot, or at any rate should not, make such a crucial difference to the outcome in law. Kennedy expects that the courts will go further towards accepting this argument, perhaps by moving in the direction already taken in Holland. He goes on to say:

> It cannot be fair to doctors to present them with a situation in which they have to guess whether people will subsequently endorse what they have done or whether, if they guess wrong, the law will be applied in all its rigour and they will face a charge of murder.[22]

Another situation is when the patient is beyond giving any kind of consent to treatment or its withdrawal. The courts dealt with one such case in 1993 (Airedale National Health Service Trust v. Bland). The patient was in what is called a persistent vegetative state and could not communicate at all. The courts decided it was lawful to stop medical treatment, including the giving of food and fluids, if in all the circumstances the patient's condition was hopeless and no benefit would be gained from any medical intervention.

The victims of degenerative diseases like Alzheimer's are not like Harold. Harold sought death because he was aware of the sharp worsening of his condition shortly before he died. He ceased to be 'himself', but not so much so that he could not say what he wished to happen, which was to die quickly. But victims of Alzheimer's are not necessarily at all aware of their state. They have ceased to be 'themselves' – lost their personalities to such an extent that they may not even have an inkling that they are dying. They cannot give consent to treatment or to its withdrawal.

So what, if anything, can be done? 'Living wills' or 'advance directives' can be of some value in other situations. They state that should you become terminally ill, you don't wish to have your life prolonged by life sustaining treatment. They are not binding on a doctor. But the BMA states that:

> The BMA strongly supports the principle of an advance directive which represents the patient's settled wish regarding treatment choices when the patient may be no longer able to completely express a view. . . . The BMA considers that a written advance directive, in the absence of contrary evidence, must be regarded as representing the patient's settled opinion.[23]

But they would not help Alzheimer's victims who, once they have the disease cannot be held to have a 'settled wish'.

The issues are so many and so tangled that there is unlikely to be a clear response to a cry like Harold's for many years to come. But a change, or set of changes, is on the way. The issue is out in the open and being widely discussed. A study reported in the *British Medical Journal*[24] (supporting the one mentioned earlier from the carer's point of view) suggested that over half of doctors had been asked to hasten a patient's death and of those 32 per cent had complied with such a request. If these results are representative, a change has already set in. Many of the doctors could be excused in law because they administered the same drugs as Dr A for relieving pain to bring on the end, but not in such a way that their intention was to speed death rather than relieve pain.

Given the gradual change in the climate of opinion, it is high time for the most stringent safeguards to be worked out and incorporated in the law. Before anything is done to aid death it must, for instance, be clear that the patient has a fatal illness and that assistance for suicide should only be given by doctors who are themselves willing to do such a thing (more maybe than were, but not all are) and who can assure themselves that the patient is completely sure about wanting death. It must also be clear that the patient is competent to take the decision, that he or she has all the necessary information on which to base it, that he or she is under no pressure at all, whether from family, doctor or the hospital, that close relatives agree to it and that the patient is free to change his or her mind.

* * *

The patients suffered physical pain. But it was not a major source of complaint, and could (without any suggestion of masochism) even produce a kind of pleasure if the level and extent of it was within their control. But the most grievous pain was not the physical; and to reduce the distress and the mental pain there is at least a case for relieving doctors from prosecution if they conform to all the necessary safeguards. This could happen, indeed is already happening to some extent, without any new legislation. The judges who have the power to modify the common law are to some extent already doing so.

Chapter 7

Beyond our care but not our caring

After the deaths of our informants, we saw as many of the carers as were willing to see us. The patients had been chosen, and chosen themselves, partly because they were willing to talk to strangers. It did not follow that the carers would be. They had not volunteered, and the last thing some of them wanted was to go back over the painful past with a stranger. So our sample was further cut down. Jennifer Barnes's husband, for instance, was not willing to see us at all after his wife's death and so we know nothing about what happened to him and his son. We were left with the carers of Donald Knight, Harold Allen, Carol Taylor, Julia Searle, Dora Anstey, Janet Rahman, Derek Wood and Kenneth Chandler. Five of these were more ready, even keener, than others to unburden themselves to us. The most detailed stories therefore come from Lilian Allen, Ivy Knight, Florence Chandler, Mrs Champion and Maria.

A great deal is already known about the subject. 'Bereavement by death is a major psychological trauma and usually takes place in the presence of members of the caring professions; consequently it has been much studied.'[1] A review of bereavement research made in 1983[2] covered more than four hundred published works. For an up-to-date tally, many more would have to be added. All we could do from our few case studies was what has not often been done before and look at the longitudinal element: the span from before to after the death and the connections between the two bereavements, the bereavement of the dying as they confronted their losses, and the bereavement of their survivors as they confronted theirs. The people who died and the people who survived were all highly individual and all the more interesting for that.

The greater grief

In at least two respects our informants were like those who have been described in other studies. They had an advantage over many other bereaved people. They all had forewarning and this, we know from the other studies, is usually a benefit denied to people who have to cope with a *sudden* death. A quick death – however much people may hope for one – is no boon for the bereaved. Parkes observed:

> Since ... the newly bereaved person is rarely able to accept, in full, the reality of what has happened, it may be that he has the same need to prepare himself for disaster as the person who has not yet experienced it. This type of anticipation has been called 'worry work' ... and when it occurs before a misfortune it has the effect of focusing the attention on possible dangers and providing an opportunity for appropriate planning. It also enables individuals to begin to alter their views of the world and to give up some of the assumptions and expectations that have been established.[3]

Our carers and patients certainly had plenty of time for worry work, and the experience of the carers was like that of the patients, both having their relatively good and their relatively bad days.

There was also a uniform rather than a variable relationship between the first bereavement and the second. Where people were mourned, the grief of the survivors was more marked than that of the dying. This is in line with previous findings. 'Despite the awe which each of us must feel in the face of death, clinical observation forces one to conclude that it is easier to die than to survive.'[4] This is barely recognised in public practice. Services are (if all goes well) mobilised for the dying. For the survivors who suffer more there is often nothing. There are ordinarily no carers for the carers in their bereavement as there were for the dying. They are on their own.

The suffering of the survivors has many components to it: the principal one is once again the pain of abandoning what Parkes calls the 'assumptive world'[5] of the bereaved which is held on to by carers even against the clearest evidence of their own eyes. It is hard enough (sometimes impossible) for the dying person to accept that he or she is going to die; that, instead of days without number, next Christmas or a wedding at Easter is the furthest to which time will stretch; and that a coming night, soon now, will be the last. But at least there is an end to it, or a presumed end, whereas the pain for the survivors can not only be very acute to start with, as they try to accept that from that sleep there will be no waking, but last for the rest of a lifetime. This was sometimes anticipated by the dying, as it was by Jennifer:

> I keep thinking about my family and feeling pain for them because I know they're going to feel a lot of pain when mine has finished. I've said to him that if he wakes up in the middle of the night and finds a shell, the shell's there but the spirit is with him. He'll have to deal with it. I feel pain for him.

Seen from outside, it beggars belief, especially in Britain, that someone who was at one time so ordinary, an ordinary wife or a not overly attached husband or another carer, should be transformed by death into an elemental creature, a figure from Greek tragedy in the streets of Bethnal Green, who draws her curtains and shuts her windows before wailing and sobbing. When she is overcome, Julia's carer, Maria, does just that: shuts all her windows and screams and shouts and hurls herself around her room; on one occasion she broke her typewriter in her anger. They seem very different from the people who went docilely in public through the motions of a funeral and disposal of the body. How is it that in private, though no longer in public, the loss can remove meaning from life and seem like the loss of all, a loss which anticipates the death in due course of the mourner and, far beyond that, of all human beings, the individual tragedy a universal tragedy, though both publicly unrecognised for what they are?

Biology no doubt plays its part as well as psychology. The fear of death, so necessary to self-preservation, is bound to have a biological base. The attachment to others must also have a similar root, essential to survival in childhood and capable of being transferred to others in adulthood.[6] But on to that root grow the attachments of a lifetime, each overlaying and drawing on the other. The relationship between the carer and the dependent invalid is bound to recall the childhood relationship of parent and child even though it is the child who has taken on the role of parent.[7] Remembering the first childhood and linking up with

the present experience of a last childhood is one of the therapeutic devices which the dying can use for themselves.

Whatever the strands that go to make up an attachment, the
cost for the mourner is grief. Rational or not, the survivors cannot
fail to feel abandoned, and experience grief as a result, grief for
themselves as well as for the person who has gone, and anger at
being abandoned. Even without these undertones and overtones
the experience would be shattering enough. The carers have to
watch and share in the gradual loss of the one capacity after
another of the dying person, and his or her grief over the loss of
the outer shell of the self. After that vicarious but painful experience, even though the physical pain is not necessarily in their
own body as well, they then have to endure the final loss on
their own account. They have to put up with the feeling that
when time stopped for the deceased, time also stopped for them.

The strain can be extreme in the period leading up to the
stopping of the clock. We can best bring this home by an account
of what it was like for one of our people. We spoke in the
previous chapter of Florence's tiredness and the controversy over
whether Kenneth should go into the hospice in order to give her
a respite. In August 1992 Kenneth eventually agreed to do this.
It was a brilliant summer and the sun was shining continually in
his first week in the hospice. He sat in his chair in the garden
every day so that he could smoke when he wanted to. Whenever
they could, Florence, her children and grandchildren sat in the
garden with him. Then a few days later Florence saw a startling
change come over him. He went very white and started, as if
seeing something strange in front of his eyes. To explain this,
Florence made a pawing movement with her curled hand in front
of her face as if trying to brush away something that was there,
and said, in Kenneth's voice – 'That black fly.' This had happened
quite often and, when she was by his side, Florence would always
brush 'it' aside. It would then disappear, momentarily swept away.
As she talked, Florence oscillated between a kind of detachment
and being very moved. The memories had been uprooted from
their place in the past and were being acted out in a continuing
and vivid present.

She had thought Kenneth was in the hospice for her sake, not
his. Then someone there said that Kenneth was not in the part
of it where patients went for a short stay – 'Oh no, Kenneth's in
the terminal'. Alarmingly, one of his daughters also overheard a

priest saying 'Kenneth, you're not afraid to die?', and him saying 'No.' What could have been chance remarks took on a much larger and more disturbing significance. Florence was therefore glad when the two weeks' stay in the hospice was up, and he came home. 'I've done my two weeks. I'm coming home now.' Florence asked, 'Did you go in just for me?' 'I did. You've got to have a break sometimes.'

Soon after his return, something miraculous happened. Kenneth had got very thin and had been eating very little in the hospice. It worried Florence more than anything. But when a daughter and her husband and children came for Sunday lunch, for once Kenneth ate a whole plateful. It was thrilling for all of them – a granddaughter got on the telephone immediately after the meal and relayed the good news to the other members of the family, house by house. The roast beef sent ripples of joy through East London. Florence always wrapped some of her own tenderness around the food she cooked for him. A little of this rubbed off on us. She had a small smile of satisfaction when we ate one of the biscuits she had ready for us to go with our cups of coffee when we arrived at the house.

It was the last time he ate like that. The only food he asked for after that was pineapple and ice-cream. It was his near death food. He asked for it on the Normandy beaches and when very ill with chemotherapy. Soon after he said, 'Please, Florence, take me to bed.' This was another shock for her. He never got out of it. A baby-sitting intercom was installed by his bed so that she could hear, magnified in the sitting room, every cough, snuffle and move. For almost three weeks he went without food, without food, without food, as Florence was apt to repeat.

He became strange in other ways too. He said, 'Florence, talk to m'mother. She's sitting next to you. What's she making all these knock-ups for? She's making loads and loads.' 'Knock-ups' were a family word for the legendary rock cakes his dead mother used to make when he was a child, and she was making them for him again. Florence would join in the make-believe, and say, 'There's enough of us here to eat them.' He would also say, 'Ronnie keeps running away from me.' Ronnie was his dead brother and Florence would join in that too and, referring to Kenneth's hand, would say, 'If I saw that hand, I'd run.' Her daughters thought Florence went too far in playing up to him and said, 'Why do you do it?' Although Kenneth spoke like that to them as well, they couldn't go along with his hallucinations as Florence did.

A little later he stopped talking in ordinary speech. Hearing being the last sense to go, he could hear them, and would smile when one of his daughters or the home nurse came into his bedroom. He would also talk by gesture. To illustrate, Florence made short cutting movements with her right hand from left to right when talking to us: it was what he did so emphatically to reject any food offered to him, cutting it to pieces before it reached him.

On his last night (as for several previous ones) he had a night nurse arranged by the hospice. Florence was sleeping on the sofa in the sitting room. The nurse woke her up in the early morning of the Monday. From the sofa Florence could see the illuminated digital clock on the oven in the kitchen. It was 5.12. She thought – 'Oh, my eyes are better. I can see the clock.' She went into the bedroom. She had a small wet sponge to clean his mouth. Kenneth wanted a cigarette. She got one and put it between two of his fingers. Florence raised her same two fingers to her mouth in a V-sign. The cigarette was never lit.

She phoned her daughter, Linda, who always drove over at 7 a.m., and asked her to come earlier. Florence told the nurse she would see a difference when Linda came in. Linda knelt and cuddled him. 'You could see the difference in him. Linda and I were in tears. The nurse said "You've got to let him go." I didn't realise how hard this was. He died not at 3.10 like on the certificate but at 3.08 on the Monday.' Florence herself was taken ill almost immediately after, more so than she'd ever been before. At times she could hardly breathe and had great sweating fits.

The final weeks were a prolonged agony for Florence, perhaps, though in a different way, even more so than for Kenneth. But she was also in one respect well prepared for what was to come. The question which all carers ask themselves is 'Could I have done more?' Hardly doubting, Florence could answer that she could not.

Florence's illnesses did not go away. They mirrored Kenneth's own troubles. Kenneth had suffered, more than anything else, from his breathing. Florence was the same and she got worse over the next two years. Her breathing spasms were most liable to attack her when she was out. 'I know he won't come back but it's a feeling that I mustn't go out.' Their daughter, Linda, also had chest problems before the anniversary of her father's death. Lilian Allen's illness was in her gut, like her husband's.

Some people would be suddenly hit in the stomach as if by a great fist, or become breathless without any apparent reason, or have tightness in the chest or a continuous dry mouth, loss of appetite, inability to sleep, exhaustion; and with these physical sensations went even more painful feelings of anger, guilt, anxiety, loneliness. All this and more has been reported before,[8] as has the length of time that it takes to go through the several stages of grief before there can be a partial recovery – from initial numbness to anger and despair and, eventually, if all goes as well as can be expected, a return to more or less normal living. But grief is not like an illness: you don't get back to normal.

Good death, bad bereavement

Terminal patients (as we said earlier) seem to last longer if they are looked after by someone who is close to them and have other people around them as well.[9] Loving care sustains and lengthens life, as one might expect, and may have played a part in the durability of three of the patients who lasted so much longer than their prognosis suggested – Kenneth Chandler (who we have just discussed), Harold Allen and Julia Searle. Harold was looked after by his wife, and Julia by her devoted friend, Maria. Maria was not a full-time carer but took a lot of time off work to be with Julia and had to do the same when she was overcome by grief after the death.

But a good death (or at least a prolonged death) for the patient may work in exactly the opposite way for the bereaved. A good death can make for a bad bereavement. The carers have had to carry the burden described in the last chapter for longer, and may have got so tired that they find it difficult to lift themselves out of it. They may also have become so intertwined with the deceased as the deceased has grown more dependent on them that, at first and for a long time afterwards, it is difficult to move towards any form of independence.

Dependence can work against a good bereavement even more powerfully than a good death – though they can of course go together. A long-term dependence can imply an insecure attachment which derives from a similar insecure attachment to parents in childhood. Chronic grief can be caused by ambivalence or ambivalent attachments.[10]

Lilian Allen was a case in point. She had been married to Harold for fifty years, and throughout it all had been dependent on her husband; he was the stronger character. She had nursed him day and night for the year he survived after his life had been given up in the hospital. She had done, and felt she had done, everything for the best.

> I've no regrets about the illness. If the time came round again I wouldn't change anything. I would still have done the same. I felt I did everything that it was possible in my power to do, at least for his last few months, because all he wanted to do was to be at home and that was made possible.

She remembered how well he had prepared for what was to come. When he was still in hospital Lilian brought in two of his relatives who had quarrelled and were not on speaking terms. She sent the two in together to see him. He talked to them and this had helped to bring them together. A rift in the family had been healed. He said: 'It was worth everything I've gone through to see them back together again as friends.' Recounting this brought tears to Lilian's eyes.

In acting like this, Harold was still very much the head of the family. He was the same when he called them all together.

> They all knew he was dying. He said to the grandchildren, 'Remember to treat your Mum and Dad the same way as they have treated us and if you follow their example you won't go far wrong.' To some of them he said they must look after me. We've all had our instructions. They often say, 'I think that's what Dad would have wanted us to do.'

She was glad he had given the instructions and that she had carried them out, about the kind of funeral he would prefer, about his choice of hymns, his laying out. We saw before how he arranged for new windows and doors in the house. He gave commands about everything. Such a one-way communication can continue and even become more insistent after death, and respect can be shown for the dead person by obeying 'to the letter' the instructions he or she gave when still alive. Last wishes can have a sacred character, and perhaps will do so even more, macabre as it will be, when dying people speak their last wishes on to video.

Harold's last weeks went fairly smoothly until near the end, and Lilian's memories of this last period – the period when, if they could, they both would have opted for euthanasia – had a nightmarish quality to them. She had to watch him stop moving, stop eating and lose weight rapidly until he began to look like the skeleton he was soon to become. She could hardly forget a moment of it. This may have been one reason she was so disturbed after his death.

She had blackouts, sometimes two or three a day. Her doctor said that for fourteen months she had been keeping herself together for Harold and the family and she had continued to do so after his death until her body could stand no more. After the giddiness had moderated, she sweated profusely and had a clammy feeling and felt sick. The blackouts, and the fear of them, kept her at home when she wanted to visit her sister. Her skin got exceedingly tender round her waist and she could not wear a skirt. At times she had agonising pains in her stomach, and could not sleep without sleeping tablets. She had terrible nightmares.

> I go out somewhere and I can't find the way home. I was in a train and couldn't find the way to Forest Gate and every time I went to ask a policeman he disappeared.

It must have been partly that she was so dependent on him. She had little to do to keep herself busy. Harold had made so many arrangements for her in his last year and her children managed the funeral. Also, she was exhausted, perhaps the most of all the carers. After that, her recovery was long drawn out. It took sixteen months before she was able to get back to a more or less ordinary life; extracts from our interview diary show this.

Early months	Lilian did not cry because Harold had asked her not to.
Four months	Lilian cries nearly the whole of every day.
Nine months	'They say it gets easier but it doesn't.'
Golden Wedding	She gave flowers to the church for the weekend of her Golden Wedding Anniversary

shortly before Christmas but could not manage to take them there herself.

Anniversary of Harold's last set-back	Lilian became more ill. Forced to see her GP; was referred to hospital.
Fifteen months	First signs of recovery. She had not been able to think of Harold except in his final months. Then she began to remember things that happened before that, like when they went in to London, 'There were flower sellers at Charing Cross station, and they always had small bunches of roses. He always bought me a bunch, *always*.'
Sixteen months	She said to herself, 'You can't go on like this forever.' After she had so clearly remembered Harold before he got ill, she began to plan for the future. She planned a holiday with her sister. During the past year she embarked on correspondence with a soldier in the Gulf. One day he paid her a surprise visit, with his girlfriend. There was a new man in her life, another soldier. Harold had left her a tape and she realised for the first time he had recorded on the second side as well. On that side he told her that she had no reason to doubt that she was right to dissuade him from becoming a professional soldier at the end of the second world war. She had often wondered whether she had been wrong. Harold had loved the army.

Maria

Maria and Julia had been friends for seventeen years and grew closer still during Julia's protracted illness. Although in a paid job herself, Maria always managed to be there when most needed. The first sign of the troubled period ahead of her was when she could not remember anything about Julia's actual death. She had been responsible for all the funeral arrangements and at the beginning this kept her very busy. Julia had told her exactly what she wanted – a dark wooden coffin with straight sides. They are very difficult to find. But Maria succeeded in finding one and, at the funeral, was congratulated by one of Julia's old hospital colleagues who had known way back that Julia had set her heart on such a coffin. There were hundreds of other things to do over the will and, when she could bear to do it, the cleaning of Julia's flat. She was in such despair that she took several months off work.

Gradually, her memories of the death came back. Julia had expressly asked her to be with her when she died. She had wanted to die at home but when the pain became uncontrollable she had to go back into hospital. Maria was with her on the last Saturday night. She had spent the whole of the previous weekend there because it was expected that Julia might die then. But this weekend there had been a slight improvement and, being very tired, Maria decided to go home to sleep. If she had had any idea what would happen she would have stayed. They both knew the day staff well and Maria thought everyone understood that she was to be called if at any time Julia took a turn for the worse.

But on this occasion the weekend night staff did not know about it. The first telephone call she had from the hospital was when the day staff came on duty. Julia died while she was rushing to the hospital. How could it have happened? Could it be that Julia had not asked for her to be called? On the Saturday night she had not wanted to talk. Maybe there was nothing more to say. Maybe she knew what was coming. But Maria's searing resentment was directed at the hospital which she felt had most miserably failed them both.

It was not until six months later that she was able to see the consultant and go over with him the whole story of Julia's last admission. She was able to say how much she felt she had let her friend down by not being there. The doctor patiently explained what had happened. The memory of that last Saturday night and the weeks leading up to it became clearer. Other memories were recovered as well. After eight months she was able to write a letter of thanks to the hospital staff for all they had done for her friend.

Another troubling question was raised by Julia's brother. He said he wished Julia could have died a year earlier, before all the pain and her three dreadful operations. Maria thought a lot about this but she most emphatically could not agree with him. The last year had been a year of 'tidying', an immense tidying of all sorts of business Julia needed to complete. She had so much to give to other people, to her nurses, to her doctors. They were all touched, and more, by her humour and her deep interest in them which was never dimmed by her suffering. Maria remembered too the precious afternoons when Julia spoke about some of her regrets, the things she felt bad about in her life. 'It seemed awful that someone should die feeling so wrong about themselves.' After they talked Julia seemed relieved. Maria felt she had been a priest and given her absolution. 'I was totally exhausted but pleased and grateful.'

Anniversaries

Throughout the first year Maria visited the grave regularly and she had the same crisis as so many other bereaved people on the anniversary of Julia's death. It was the culmination of a stressful year. She had had irritable bowel syndrome before and it flared up after Julia's death. She found herself in hospital for tests, watching other radiographers use on her the equipment Julia had once used on others. Later on she began to fear the coming anniversary of the death, wondering why the thought seemed to take up so much of her energy and for so long a time. The anniversary that mattered was not the same date in the calendar, which fell on Monday, but the Sunday immediately before. Julia had died on a Sunday. She visited Julia's grave then. Up until then Maria had been able to say to herself 'I was doing this with Julia last year at this time.' The anniversary made that impossible.

I didn't want it to come ... to be able to say that Julia had been dead for a year. I didn't want to pass through it.

Lilian had many of the same physical symptoms as others. But the pains in her stomach (she sometimes felt she spent the whole day on the toilet) were more serious and got so bad that nine months after Harold's death she was sent for tests to the same hospital she (and Dr Clayton) had once rescued him from. There was no cancer but she was told to return for further tests in January. Christmas was coming. It was the blackest period she had. There was Christmas to brace herself for and Harold's birthday at the end of December and the anniversary of his death on New Year's Day.

The day before New Year's Eve Harold had gone into a coma and it was the last day she had spoken with him. The next day was his birthday and she read his birthday cards to him. 'It'll be years before I forget New Year's Eve.' Lilian relived every minute of it and got more ill as she did. She called the wonderful GP to visit her on New Year's Day. He was very upset she had got so poorly without telling him.

Florence's daughter made her go to her GP a week or so before the anniversary because she was in increasing pain with her breathing. The GP was cross with her, as he had been before for her smoking, and said 'I want you to have an x-ray immediately.' Florence hovered but, under pressure, agreed to go to the hospital that same afternoon. There was no cancer, but there was severe congestion. Linda, the eldest daughter, got a chest infection at the same time.

Florence was well enough to visit the cemetery on the anniversary day and shortly afterwards took down from the place where it had been a small card with Kenneth's picture on it. It had kept falling over in the breeze from the open window. Every time this happened the girls said 'daddy's here'. It was too much for Florence. She put the card in a drawer. Shortly after the anniversary, the GP was called again. Her chest infection was worse. Her cough 'starts as soon as you put your head on the pillow', as it had with her husband.

Ivy

Donald was not one of those who lived so much longer than the prognosis. But in other respects Ivy was similar to Lilian Allen and to Maria in the care she had given. One of her problems was the same as Maria's. Maria was worried by Julia having to go into hospital, Ivy by Donald going into the hospice. The home nurse had suggested it, and his sister sanctioned it, otherwise she would not have agreed. Donald was deteriorating, becoming less than the man she knew; he and she were at the end of their tether. So she was both relieved, and guilty for being relieved, even though she recognised that the hospice had eased his last two weeks. 'I thought "this is practical Christianity".'

Her failure to be there at the death was even more upsetting

and, unlike Maria, it was more her responsibility. She did not
start wondering about it until three months into her bereavement.
Should she have stayed with Donald on the evening he died?
She had been there all day. The hospice staff had asked her to
stay because they thought he would die soon; but she did not.
When she remembered it all, she was left with the rankling
question, even two years after the death, should she not have
come home? The staff said he did not open his eyes. 'But I'm
wondering if he opened his eyes and I wasn't there.'

She also worried because they had never talked together about
his having cancer. Soon after his death Ivy demonstrated with a
clenched fist her sense of having been right not to tell Donald.
But her certainty gradually dissolved. Did he know about it, or
not? She eventually decided that he did. When the home nurses
came from St Joseph's he leant over on his pillow and said, 'I
suppose that's where I shall end up.' Ivy dismissed this quickly
saying, 'Oh, don't let's have you talking like that.' She decided
he did not say any more because he thought that she did not
want to talk about it. It was painful to go over again.

Her outward show concealed all these doubts and reflections.
At the funeral she started out in the way she intended to continue.
Her nephew expected everyone to be crying but she would have
none of it.

We don't do that. The time for crying is on your own. I did
all my crying when he was ill. I think you owe it to people
who support you not to break down. It's bad form. My mum
did cry at Dad's funeral but only in the car.

She also restrained herself when she was on her own.

Crying is nothing but self pity. I've felt the need for tears but
fought it. They'll bring me down.

But it was only show. The physical pain of it – 'it hits you in
the solar plexus' – was added to spiritual pain. She had to turn
away when she saw a couple in the street, her nostalgia was so
sharp. She had to turn off the radio when an old tune he liked
was played. She could not even face their bedroom. Her tactic was
to distract herself by keeping very busy. She cleared out all his
clothes, had a surplus storage tank removed to create space,
arranged for the flat to be decorated and began to consider
installing central heating.

I keep myself busy. I had so many things to do one day, sorting out my papers and everything and then when it was done I stopped, paused and wondered, what now? My stomach turned over inside me and I was physically sick. What I feel is bereft.

Taking a holiday in Scotland was part of distracting herself. But when she got off the bus and wondered at the splendour of the view, she said, 'Oh look Don!' She often thinks, 'Oh I'll tell Don that.'

* * *

It was somewhat easier for people who had companions. As Ivy said, 'I've wanted someone I could talk to. People think you don't want to talk, but you need it.' In this crisis of their lives most people needed a community, or at least some people who would, in small ways at least, care for them as they had cared for the deceased. It was also partly that they wanted someone to listen to the almost endless repetition of their accounts of the fatal illness, without saying 'You must pull yourself together now – you can't mope like this for ever.'

The sense of futility could not be avoided. 'I was totally over-whelmed,' said Maria. 'The whole of me was crying with despair and with the loss and futility of it all.' Is there any point in anything when a life that seemed so meaningful was snuffed out so easily? The answers that are most convincing come not in the form of answers but as affirmations of the ordinary world made up of tens of thousands of individual and collective habits, modes of actions and thought that are taken for granted, even if it is awful that the ongoing world does not contain the deceased. Only relatives, neighbours, friends and acquaintances can bring back that ordinary world and one of the best hopes of recovery is for the bereaved, when the time comes, to make overtures to it and the people in it. But it is not easy. Fear of death, the uncertainty about how to deal with it, and embarrassment about what to say, tells against the very sympathy which the bereaved need so badly.

The grief shown by the principal carers was in many ways similar to that described before. They went through the same sort of stages and had to face up to the same contradictions. Death hits at the heart of familiar habits generated over many years. It arouses the perennial fears of abandonment. It removes much of the meaning of ordinary daily activities. The meaning is the shared meaning, which only stands up as long as it is not questioned. Once questioned, it can seem nothing is there, a void. Everything can, to use Maria's word again, seem 'futile'.

Here in a different form is the ancient railing against God for allowing all this suffering. What are we struggling for if it all comes to nothing, if the mourners will soon come to the same end, raising the same disturbing questions? Death raises doubt about individual emotions and also about communal existence, for it is from communal existence that the values come which (when they are shared) help to give meaning to the individual life. In an individualistic society, people are left to get on with their grief work largely on their own, sometimes constrained by the belief of those like Ivy who think that by hiding their sorrow away they are showing the proper spirit.

If a good death is followed by a hard bereavement, can anything be said about ways to mitigate it? Not that there was much in the way of choice. Where the carers loved the dying, they were glad they could care for him or her, and would not have had it otherwise. They knew that the suffering was the price of their love, and would not have that otherwise either. They were going through an experience which, however frightful it was, had its illumination as well. They learnt more about themselves; they learnt more about life through being so close to death.

The dying could also help the bereaved by returning the love so that it remained a comfort after the death, and as real (or almost as real) as it had been in life. The person who dies in peace, with acceptance rather than bitterness, bestows a gift upon the survivors which lasts for them, and can quieten their own fears. The dying can also help by as far as possible encouraging the carers to retain a certain measure of independence.

But recovery is a relative term. Few of these people will be the same again. They will never forget what has happened nor completely put their grief to rest. We said that the company of others can help. But the general community, so much in evidence at death in some other cultures, was not apparent in the same way for most of our people. They did not live in the idealised English community of Ambridge where everybody knows everybody. Community support was, despite all its shortcomings, visible enough in the period before the death. The Home Care nursing service was testament to that. For cancer sufferers, the hospices have produced wonderful opiates. But for the spiritual pain of the dying or of the mourners, what can be done for that? The question brings us on to the subject of the next chapter, the afterlife.

Chapter 8

The afterlife

We have been describing the manner in which some of the bereaved managed less to work through than to 'pain through' their ordeal after the death; and now want to mention one of the comforts which could bring some relief. Kenneth, Donald, Julia and the rest were dead, or at any rate their bodies were. But after death an afterlife could restore them to a kind of life which could be both reassuring and (at times) disturbing.

They became ghosts, or spirits, or manifestations of the deceased. Ghost beliefs are almost universal in human societies. In a comparative study, ghost beliefs were found to be present in sixty-five out of sixty-six societies for which there was written information.[1] Many of the accounts of particular societies are classics. 'At death the soul becomes a ghost (*nyaakpiin*), which, like an errant soul, is visible at certain times to certain people; only after the shrine has been created at the final ceremony does it become a spirit proper (*kpiin*).'[2] 'They are almost completely devoid of any fear of ghosts, of any of these uncanny feelings with which we face the idea of a possible return of the dead.'[3] 'Apparitions of the dead were especially common in the period immediately after a death i.e. when the emotional sense of loss was most keen and presumably the tendency to visualize the form of the departed most vivid.'[4] And so on.

In all the sixty-five societies there was no hiding away of ghost beliefs. The difference in modern conditions is that the apparitions are not alarming and that the bereaved believe in them and the people around them, bound into a rationalist culture, do not, or at any rate strongly affect not to do so. This can help to separate off the deceased from ordinary people, increase the stress on the bereaved and sometimes go as far as to make them fear they are going out of their minds,[5] when what they are going through is a very common experience. It would be nearer the truth to say that it is the unfeeling majority who are 'mad'.

For some people the dead can be a greater comfort than the living. The dead can be summoned at any time. They do not have to be telephoned in advance for an appointment. They can be a great solace for older people who are terminally ill, bereaved and still mourning spouses. The marriage service gets it wrong when it says 'Till death us do part.' Death is not necessarily a parting. The older were expecting to die, but unlike the others in the sample who were hoping that they would not, they hoped, on the contrary, that they would, and soon, so that the parting would not last. With few still-alive people to be so much attached to,[6] they created another world from which their departed had not departed, and – this being the beauty of it – a world into which they too could enter through the gateway of death and so be re-united with those they continued to love as much as ever.

Alice did not feel a great need for friends in this life partly because she was looking forward so much to being with her one true friend again. She spoke of 'going up to see Dad', her husband. In this she was like some of the younger people. Janet said:

> When you die you meet with your family members. They will be waiting for me. I sometimes see my Mum when I go to bed at night and I say goodnight. I will meet up with my Mum, Dad and Nan.

Other people had no wish to die but had some comfort from expecting to join those who had already died. Kenneth was also sure he would rejoin his dear dead mother and brother who had kept him going through all his illnesses, and even taken away his pain. When he said that 'a family is the real pleasure of life' he meant the members of the family who were dead as well as those still alive. He interviewed his dead relatives regularly. Sitting down in his favourite chair, after Florence had gone to bed, he would be by himself with the comforting ghosts whom he could so effectively conjure up from the dead.

> Without their help I wouldn't be here to talk to you. They've carried me through the heart trouble and the cancer. If I'm going through extraordinary discomfort I say 'give me your help'. Every evening I go to them and I talk to them. I talk

to them together. The ones I pick out are Mum and Ron. I thank them for their help during the day and for looking after me during the night. Wthout their help, I wouldn't have got to where I am today. I get a great feeling of relief. I really feel they are here helping me.

Our informants did not bring out the kind of accounts of the afterlife which Gorer[7] recorded some thirty years before, when one widow was presumably reflecting her own experience when she said there will be 'no sex in heaven' and another woman thought the afterlife would be in a 'place where we don't worry about money'. A widower in the rainy south-west expected that in the new world he would go to it would always be daylight and 'the sun always shines'. A shopkeeper in Scotland believed not so much in an afterlife as an after-existence of another sort. 'The stars we see above are people who have gone before us shining down.' But many of Gorer's informants were far less specific than that, considering the future after death as a mystery – in this being with St Paul:

> Eye hath not seen nor ear heard, neither have entered into the heart of man, the things which God hath prepared for them that love Him.
>
> (I Corinthians 2: 9)

The people in our sample were more limited. They spoke, almost exclusively, about their dead relatives.

Looking forward to the reunion

Many of our people were hoping to join their relatives. A cemetery not far away provided plenty of evidence to the same effect, of people waiting to be re-united. The crematorium was in the middle of a garden of remembrance. The garden was criss-crossed by walkways. On their kerbs were brass plates behind which the ashes of a dead person had been strewn in the shape of a cross until the rain sank them into the grass or the wind blew them away. The brass plates all had inscriptions on them and some of these bore messages to assure someone who had already died that the parting was only temporary; FOR ARTHUR MILLS UNTIL WE MEET AGAIN – HIS JEANIE; or FOR JIM WHILE WE ARE PARTED FROM SALLY BARROW.

Many of the plates had had further inscriptions added to them
by children or other relatives after a second death. The further
inscriptions were all about the joy of being re-united with loved
ones, like these three examples.

BETTY VINEY
TOGETHER AGAIN
WITH HUSBAND JOE

TOGETHER AGAIN
RE-UNITED IN ETERNITY
TOGETHER AT LAST
VERA AND TOM SARSON

LOVINGLY RE-UNITED
LOVED ALWAYS
LILY JEBB   BOB JEBB
4/1/1988   4/5/1994

Another cemetery had the same little plaques under the small
rose trees planted around the crematorium and graves nearby as
well. On a Christmas Day it was full of people who had come to
bring presents to their dead. The adults mostly had flowers laid
for them and the children cards or more ordinary presents. A
boy was in the same grave as his dad and grandad. Hanging on
a cross of fresh flowers was a large card saying 'Billy. For a
Special Boy on his Birthday. 2.' Another child's grave was piled
high with toys inside transparent bags to protect them from the
weather – a toy Porsche, a Jaguar, a fire-engine, a carton of
chocolate with a card 'From a loving dad, grandad, great-
grandad.'

Phantoms

The prospect of reunion with the dead was not immediate. It
could not happen until the living were themselves dead, and for
this happy outcome people had to wait. But it did not mean that
in the interim there was nothing for them to do except wait with
what patience they could muster. The dead could not be shuffled
off somewhere else where they also had nothing to do except
wait for their relatives to rejoin them. The dead were waiting,
but also very much a presence in the lives of the people they

were waiting for. Parkes described widows one year after the
death.

These memories were remarkable for their clarity. The dead
person would be pictured exactly as when he was alive. Usually
he would be 'seen', for instance, in his accustomed chair, and
the memory would be so intense as almost to amount to a
perception: 'I keep seeing his very fair hair and the colour of
his eyes'; 'I still see him, quite vividly, coming in the door.'[8]

The behaviour has also been observed in other social animals
who 'search' for what is lost.[9] Phantom husbands and wives have
been noticed as much as phantom limbs[10] in other societies, and
of course in other religions. In Japan 'Shintoism and Buddhism
both encourage the living to maintain a sense of relatedness to
the dead, and even to discuss the events of the day with the dead
at a family altar.'[11]

Shintoism and Buddhism are not common in East London. But
the behaviour was not so different. No sooner is the coffin closed
than people can encounter the dead person again. It can hardly
be otherwise when the dead have left behind so many reminders
of themselves, and any of the reminders can be so vivid as to
recall the dead to life. One ever-present reminder was emptiness,
the dead house empty of sound, or any space which had not been
empty before. It is common enough in ordinary life to treat
objects in space as though they are people – the chair that a
person sat in before leaving a meeting is turned to when the
person is mentioned later on as though he or she were still there
and their empty chair can hear. Downing Street is worried, the
White House is angry, Paris is friendly towards Bonn. In the same
way it is impossible not to look at the empty chair or empty bed
which the dead person used to occupy and see him or her in it
again, or the pillow without a head on it. Lilian would reach out
in the middle of the night 'to touch Harold'. Kenneth's chair
stood empty throughout the family Christmas gathering so that
everyone would be aware of him.

The emptiness is sacrosanct. No-one else should be in the bed
or use the pillow or sit in the chair. Even young children can feel
the embargo. Harold's $2\frac{1}{2}$ year old grandson was very insistent
that no-one should sit in his grandpa's chair when his parents
brought him to visit, nor drink from his grandpa's mug. In such
circumstances it may be impossible not to feel empty yourself. 'I

am absolutely empty,' said Derek's friend, Mrs Litten. 'I'm not lonely. I'm empty. When he was here he filled me.'

People could be most at one with the dead when they were in the house of the dead, and, for this reason, several of the mourners did not want to go out at all. They could behave there as they had always done, in East London as has been reported elsewhere. With much larger numbers than ours 'Fifty-two percent of our sample refused to modify some practice that would acknowledge their husband's deaths; for example, they continued to set a place for them at dinner or they cooked as much food as they had when the husband was alive.'[12] It was almost as if they were entombed together; if they left home they wanted to get back to it again as soon as they could. If they went on a little holiday, or to stay with a relative, they could not wait to get back early, and it was a relief when they did. As soon as Lilian opened her front door she called to Harold that she was back. Ivy talked all the time to Donald's photograph on the top of the television.

Maria did not live with Julia. But she used to phone her in the evenings, and when that customary time came around there was a pang when she thought, 'My God I'll never call her again.' But Julia's flat was nearby and when Maria passed by on her way home at night she would look up to the windows half-expecting the light to be on. When there was no light, she wondered whether if she went up there she would still find Julia sitting alone in the darkness. She did go in sometimes with the key she had kept and always hunted for a message from Julia. It was the message she might have got if she had been at her bedside when she died. She also wondered, when she was there, whether Julia was watching her. 'I say to her "if you are here watching me, show me by moving something".' One day she was pleased that one of the pictures in the hall was hanging askew as though someone had twisted it round. Mrs Champion was much comforted by a 'message' she found from Carol. It was a Christmas card from a previous year which she'd forgotten, saying 'Thank you for everything. I couldn't have managed without you.' Mrs C thought nothing of it when she'd first received it. But rediscovered, it had the utmost significance, being regarded as a message from the dead.

The comfort and the pain

The communion with the dead was always double-edged. On the one hand it was a comfort, partly because the dead person was, for all of the people for most of the time, thought of as benign, not as the hostile and terrifying ghost, reported in other cultures, who want the living to join them post-haste. For Ivy Knight and Lilian Allen the communication was reassuring. Ivy talked to Donald almost continuously, even when watching Coronation Street which they used to watch together, and it made her cry so much she had to switch it off.

> I talk to him when I dust or I just tell him what I'm going to do, like I'm going to bed now because I don't want to watch the TV. I don't go to the cemetery. He's here, all round me, all the time, he's not there.

This did not mean she did not want to visit the cemetery. But Don had asked her not to. When one day she could not resist going she got as far as the gates, 'I can hear his voice and I think I'm breaking faith if I go in there. The only reason I stopped was Don's voice saying to me "you won't go there by yourself, will you?", and I promised.' Nearly a year after Donald's death, when she was thinking of getting rid of a table in the kitchen because she wanted to install central heating and there wasn't room for the table any more, she spoke to him about it.

> I can hear you telling me, love, you made it, but it'll have to go. I need the space.

She consulted him about anything to do with the house, even if not always taking his advice. Perhaps not taking it made him more real.

> He's part of me, with me. When that man gave me the quote of £300 for decorating the room – when he'd gone I looked at Don's photograph and said 'that's a bit steep'.

Harold, too, is with his wife in the house. She says 'Harold is here'.

> I've woken up around 6 o'clock and seen Harold's side of the bed empty and thought 'Oh, where is he? He must be up already and downstairs', and slowly I've come round and realise he's not there. . . . I often think, oh I'll ask Harold,

and then think, no you can't. Perhaps people who've had more separate lives don't find it so difficult.

When she dozes in the sitting room and wakes and he's not there she again thinks, 'I expect he's making a cup of tea.'

Mrs Litten did not so much talk to her partner as have a powerful sense of a presence.

> I come in here sometimes and I feel a presence in the room. It's uncanny. It's like the whole room being filled with him.

It was the same with Mrs Champion, except she talked to her daughter as well.

> I go out in the garden at night and Diane says why? I say 'your Mam's here'. I speak to her when I come in as well. She would be there in the kitchen waiting, bald, with her little turban on, and I say 'hello', and talk to her.

So also with Kenneth. One night, a daughter, Christine, brought around a poem written some time before by her husband about what Kenneth was like with Christine and the others when they were children. Christine put the poem in a brown envelope on top of the fridge. Florence said:

> We were in the kitchen talking about Dad and this poem was sitting on top of the fridge and there was no window open and it floated across my head and on to the table in front of me. 'Mum, Daddy's here,' I said 'Yes, I know.'

Earlier a copy of the poem had been put into Kenneth's coffin, along with a set of family photographs. One of his girls went to the crematorium regularly to talk to Kenneth and continued to seek his advice as though he was still alive. Sixteen months after the death Linda was still going weekly to the cemetery where the ashes were interned. She washed the gravestone every time she went, talked to him and did not fail to tell him what had happened in the week since she was there last. Nearly two years after the death she had a stone heart made to go with the headstone. Her heart was not like that. The daughters continued to summon him to maintain order. When one of his daughters was cross with her daughter for the mess she was making she said, 'Grandad's watching you.' Not unsurprisingly, the grand-daughter turned the tables on her mother on another occasion

when she did not like what her mother was doing by also saying,
'Grandad's watching you.'

Pulling the other way

On the other hand, however comforting the memories of the
dead person, especially when they go beyond memory and take
shape as a voice or a sense of a presence,[13] the same experiences
are always on the balancing edge between consolation and
despair. The bereaved in our study were perfectly well aware, at
any rate when disbelief could not be suspended, that the dead
are dead; imagining it not so could then add greatly to the poign-
ancy. The empty chair in which for a moment he might seem to
be sitting was really (and the word still meant something) empty,
the voice was not really hers, he could not really admire the view
with you. The hallucination could point up the awful contrast
between the imagined and the actual. It has really happened. The
dead person has gone – is not making the tea or twisting the
picture on the wall. A hope is continually turning into the sadness
of hope against hope. Because in imagination he or she is right
there with you, looking and sounding the same as ever, his or
her actual and complete absence can be all the more bitterly
painful.

We saw the same kind of ambivalence about the dead person's
possessions, which in this situation *are* the dead person – above
all their clothes. They represented the dead most especially when
they were hanging up in a way which almost looked like the
person who had once been inside them. They were regarded,
and guarded, by Kenneth's daughters as more than mere outer
garments. For fear that their mother would dispose of them they
took many of the clothes away. One daughter went off with some
of his shirts, another with one of his suits to hang in her wardrobe,
another took his metal leg with the hole in it which had so
intrigued children and grandchildren. His aftershave had to
remain on the bath so that the children could make sure it was
still there when they came to visit. When Florence threw away
his comb there was 'uproar' on the part of the daughters. The
bathroom was part of the family shrine, and nothing was to be
touched. Their mother was less keen on keeping intact objects
which also had such painful associations. She had to take his old

shoes away secretly when no-one was there and without telling the guardians what she had done.

For a long time Maria could not give away any of Julia's clothes. They were so stylish and so much an expression of her personality. Nor could she go, without crying, near D.H. Evans where Julia had bought most of the clothes in the first place. Mrs Champion went to live in Carol's home six months before her death. She stayed on to look after Carol's daughter and slept in Carol's bedroom but for eight months after her death could not take any of Carol's clothes out of the wardrobe or the drawers. Mrs Champion's clothes remained in suitcases on the floor. Ivy packed up Donald's clothes in a fit of anger but found it difficult giving them away. If he came back, he would need them.

A family religion

The belief in an afterlife was taken to its fullest extent in the first year or so after the death when the anguish was greatest and the need for a balm most acute. As the sorrow lifted a little, Lilian's memory of the death became a little less sharp, time which had stopped began to move again and she was able to remember back to the good, to the ordinary times when her husband bought red roses for her from the flower seller at Charing Cross Station. Harold too became a bit less of an immediate presence in her life. It was the same with Maria when she remembered the fun she had enjoyed with Julia. She did not look up so often when passing to see if Julia's light was on. This is not to say that any of the bereaved who had suffered severely ever, or would ever, consider that their dead were completely gone. They were in an afterlife into which in their turn the bereaved would one day enter.

There was little indication that people in general had got their belief in the afterlife from their church. This was despite the fact that they mostly considered themselves as being attached to a church – of the patients four were Catholic, seven Anglican, one Jewish, two were of no religion – of the bereaved, six were Anglican, one Catholic, one Muslim. A few of the patients were visited weekly by priests and given communion at home. Some of them preferred a belief in an afterlife which arose directly out of their religion. But all that was different from the feelings they were now having of the dead being still alive, indeed so alive that they could be 'seen' and 'heard'. Most did not think

of the experiences they were now having in their encounters with
the dead as being in any way the same as those that were featured
in church. The link was not there, except for Carol.

I believe you go somewhere. Where I don't know. I believe
you go on to God. I believe there is a heaven. If the time is
up, I've got to know there is something beyond, something
that makes it worthwhile, that it's not all been in vain.

But for the most part their religion was of a private and personal
kind. Love was as central to it as in formal religion. Only if they
loved the person who had died would they have faith in that person's continued life. If pressed, they might have been persuaded

And now abideth faith, hope, charity, these three; but the
greatest of these is charity.

(I Corinthians 13: 13)

But they did not take their ideas directly from the Bible; even if
they knew that charity means love, they did not necessarily know
that love is the necessary condition of the belief in a kind of
afterlife. It is only those who are loved who seem to live on, and
the faith and hope is that they are doing so.

But their religion was a family religion, since it was mostly a
dead member of a family or quasi-family who was thought to be
waiting for the family to be re-united and re-formed. They did
not have general ideas about resurrection. But they had a notion
of heaven: it was a place where they would be united with those
they loved who also loved them, in which there would presumably
be no room for those who loved no-one. But it was heaven
divided, as though it was a dark but infinitely large cathedral
made up of countless small chapels in which families could join
up as they had been on earth. It was a religion having its source
not so much in general teachings as in the primordial psychology
of loss and of the manner in which loss of the gravest sort is
dealt with. This is the stuff from which religions are made.

This means, as we see it, that folk beliefs about the afterlife of
a most fundamental kind are liable to be out of harmony with
the theology and practice of the churches. It was notable how
rare it was for people to make a connection between any orthodox notion of their church, or any church, about the afterlife and
their own view of it. Their private religious views were not linked
in any ostensible way to institutional ones.

There was a gap between private and public religion. It was as though the churches, to which people belonged in a very nominal way and still made use of for funerals, had pulled in one direction and their members in another. The main influence has been the same. The general secularisation of society, which has (if we are right) been accompanied by a lay view of immortality, has penetrated the church itself through a thousand windows, sapping religious confidence and undermining religious conviction; it has also thinned down the beliefs that lay people have inherited from a long tradition and left them to wander around, in this small group or that, with their own beliefs or lack of them. Until they became housebound, people who were confident about an after-life (but not confident enough to noise it abroad lest they make fools of themselves) were on a Sunday morning less likely to be at church than at the supermarket in order to make sure that at any rate this life was well provided for.

* * *

The most striking feature of the accounts recorded in this chapter was the manner in which the dead person seemed to manifest himself or herself (always retaining a gender in death) in life. Not by deliberate decision, sometimes indeed in spite of them-selves, people reasserted the denial of death (which Dr Kübler-Ross made so much of when referring to the dying) which had apparently been surrendered in face of the actual death. This same behaviour has been described more vividly by anthropol-ogists in studies of pre-literate societies. The descriptions of their psychological state given by our people are very similar. In this respect, under our clothes and even under our skins, we are all, apparently, like each other. But the psychological need for sup-port from others is not satisfied in the same way as in some other places. In an individualistic society, people are left to get on with their grief work largely on their own, sometimes constrained by the illusion of those like Ivy who think that by hiding their sorrow away they are showing the 'good form' of which the community approves and which is so much a matter of pride. Without much in the way of wider collective support the family exerts its influ-ence again. The presence of family and family substitutes helps the dying towards a good death; the combined presence of dead relatives helps the grieving towards a good bereavement.

Chapter 9

In conclusion: collective immortality

As engaged bystanders, we have been trying to convey some sense of what it was like to be dying and mourning. At a particular moment in the general history and in their own, the people were going through the same sort of experience that all of us, unless we die on the instant, are likely to have.

The two forces driving the current changes in the way people die are the state of medicine and the influence of individualism, each sharing with all religions and legal codes the principle that life (but not death?) is sacred. Cancer is no longer as swift a killer as it was, and because the victims of cancer and many other maladies are living longer, more people are alive who know they are going to die soon enough for them to be very aware of its imminence. More of the living are dying; the greater numbers have given them greater prominence. The need to care for them has given rise to the new institutions of hospices, home nurses and the like, and has helped to encourage bereavement counselling. But there is a great deal more to do to satisfy new sets of needs which are already urgent, and will grow steadily. Death is already being more written about and discussed. Death is no longer taboo.

Individualism, the other main influence, not only embraces hedonism and self-seeking generally, it also takes in the assertion of new rights for the individual in the face of authority. The authority of doctors to do what they like, and to maintain their power inviolate by keeping quiet about it, has been brought increasingly under question. The resulting openness has made possible a new kind of good death for more people. The same influences may be at work to bring about new kinds of funeral in which more is made of the individual who has died.

We do not see any reason to think that these two major, interlinked influences will wither away, or that the associated trends in behaviour have yet run their course. The question we are raising is whether the first set of influences, to do with medicine, is going to underpin a much more momentous change in the attitude towards death itself. Is death going to be transformed again? We have been persuaded that it probably will, and we will come back to that a little later in this chapter after we have taken stock of our findings.

The goodness of the patients

Even allowing for the compensations which may be gained from its slow progress, cancer has to be reckoned a wretched disease, both to have and to care for. But we are less impressed by the misery of our people than we are by the fortitude with which most of them (especially the older) suffered it, their calmness of bearing, their courage and their goodness. Although to some limited extent they may have been on their best behaviour with us as their memorialists, it is hard to believe that people so near to death, their own or another's, would go to any great lengths to put on a special performance, or, insofar as they were doing so, keep up a deception week after week, month after month, in some cases year after year. Much of what they were was what we saw and heard, and from what we saw and heard in this extremity the goodness stood out. It was a tribute to them as well as to death for the qualities it brings out.

The goodness was more obvious for people who died a social death, when those they were close to were near them, and especially for those who had a generally harmonious relationship with their kin, or, more remarkably, with people who became substitutes for kin. The good that people do lasts after them: it certainly lasts, and on the whole to their benefit, through a long illness. Insofar as the book has been a search for the good death, the first somewhat anodyne conclusion has to be that a good death emerges from a good life.

But there is obviously more to it than that as there is also more to it than that pain should be controlled in the lead-up to death. There seems to be at work around death a peculiar and harsh principle of justice. People with permanent and loving relationships, which sustain them wonderfully through their illness and death, have more to lose, and their survivors too. Their fortune can also be their misfortune. People who are not so sustained can find it easier to die: they have less to lose, and maybe more to hope for. This is a secular version of the old rule that the more a person suffered in this life, the more he or she would be rewarded in the next. Looked at like this, a good dying implies more heartache for the dying and even more so for the bereaved. Death is the supreme loss. Pain is the sacrifice that love imposes, especially on the survivors. Any consideration of a good death has to take in more than the death itself, and extend beyond it.

There is no let up for those who have carried the burden through many long days and many longer nights. They have to watch death take its slow and relentless course. While this is happening, it is difficult for both the carers and the cared for to keep hope flickering, but perhaps more so for the carers. The carers can see what is happening while the dying can more readily have recourse to that inner self somewhere inside them which is untouched by the disease. The carers may also have to put up with a conflict of interest in themselves and between themselves and their patients.

However long-drawn-out the illness, the patients who are being looked after usually want it to be still more extended; and so, generally, do the carers. But, however much they push the thought away from them, carers are liable to be more divided about it, hoping to be released from their burdens, and hoping also they will not. The carers (as well as the dying) are apparently able to call on almost miraculous powers of endurance on behalf not of self-preservation but of other-preservation. But these powers can be put to such a test that they are brought to the point of collapse. The 1963 Institute study on the mortality of widowers showed that. One death can precipitate another.[1] The fight against death can be so strenuous as to incapacitate others.[2] Heroes can have their victims by their side. 'In adult life recent studies have implicated bereavement in the causation of several types of cancer: Idiopathic Glossodynia; Cushing's Syndrome and oral lichen planus.'[3] Unless extraordinarily insensitive, the dying know what their carers are going through. So the more that can be done to help the carers, the better it is for the dying.

Support for the carers

The carers have voluntarily, and usually knowingly, brought misery and strain on their own heads. The carers, without the love which made them willing to go to such lengths, even to risk a kind of suttee for themselves, would not have undergone the same strain or the same misery. They – or anyone willing to endure as much on behalf of others – demonstrate that love is not love if it cannot bear misery. They are, by acting as they do, upholding the values that make something of a community out of a society; they are renewing the reservoir of goodwill from which anyone may need to draw at any time. A Jewish proverb urges you to repent on the day before you die. It can also be said – give something to others on the day (and days) before you die, the more so if you get nothing obvious in return. It can be the way to satisfy 'the spectator within the breast', 'the great judge and arbiter of their conduct' inside everyone, to use the words of Adam Smith, who was a philosopher[4] as well as an economist. It was notable in our study that several of the carers, as they moved towards recovery, thought they had learned a great deal from their bereavement – had 'grown' through it.

On a more mundane level carers are also, even if they get an attendance allowance, unpaid nurses saving taxpayers money by looking after people who would otherwise have to be more expensively maintained in and out of institutions. If it were not for these nurses, the slowing down of death could by now have caused a financial crisis even more severe than anything the National Health Service has had to face so far. Already NHS expenditure per head for people aged 75 and over is more than four times that for the population as a whole.[5] It could be much worse; a host of taxpayers could have joined the euthanasia lobby. In their role of unpaid nurse, the unpaid carers therefore deserve support. They should be but are not the beloved of the Treasury.

Regard the carers as nurses and it is clear what some of their needs are. As much as most of the patients, they cry out for honesty, which we presented in Chapter 5 as a primary need. If doctors try to conceal the fact of the disease, or fail to explain what is happening as it unfolds, it is even more blameworthy than if they do the same to paid nurses. If they make the family into accomplices in a lie, they can add horribly to the misery. Ignorance can augment fear, with imagination adding to torment and, perhaps worst of all, distrust be introduced into the vital web of relationships around the patient. We don't pretend it is easy to be honest if pains are taken to avoid being brutal about it. Honesty driven by respect for the person takes more time and trouble than dishonesty devoid of that respect. Once stated, the case for taking the time and the trouble almost makes itself.[6]

These nurses are untrained as well as unpaid. If honesty is one need, another, more wide-ranging, is for skilled support. To carry them through, they need someone to hand, in person and on the phone, to whom they can turn for information and advice in all the trials and emergencies which the dying and their carers are heir to. If they do not know what they should do for the best, or fear they will be caught out alone when faced with a crisis, that can itself be one of the most severe strains of all, and even the reason why they give up.

The nursing services

All our patients and carers were fortunate in having the home nursing service to call on. When Kenneth, in virtue of the fact that he could already boast four dutiful and loving daughters, named the Home Care nurse his Number Five Daughter, he was voicing the sentiments of many of our people. After their initial terror of admitting these angels of death into their homes, they grew to welcome them more and more warmly. A nurse trained to help dying people, with skilled back-up for their carers, frequently becomes, even though only for a short period, a friend of the family. She or he can offer so much of the right kind of support that a service as good as St Joseph's needs to be made available as soon as possible to cover the whole country. Much of East London, so disadvantaged in other ways, is in this respect privileged.[7]

GPs, too, can be immensely valuable; or they can be a running irritant if they steer well clear of their dying patients. But even where doctors are able to visit, there is still a need for nurses to be on call, visit more frequently and bring to the afflicted what only skilled nursing can bring. It would be an advantage for both nurses and GPs if they had more respite beds available for patients on a temporary basis. A couple of weeks' rest can be a life-saver for a harassed carer – who, without a break, could be at the end of her or his tether. Any support of that kind can aid the elusive good death.

But as far as the policy and effort of the National Health Service is concerned, we would put most emphasis on the need for an expansion of Home Care for people who are dying so that present regional and local inequalities can be reduced, and more people in more places (and not just sufferers from cancer) get the benefit of the kind of home service which was available to our patients. No act of policy could do more than that to add to the numbers of people who have a relatively good death. A majority of people (as we noted in Chapter 4) would prefer not just to be looked after at home over the period of the illness but to die at home. Home nursing support makes this more possible for more people, reduces the number of people who have to suffer the pain of dying in a place in which they don't want to be and allows more carers to be beside people when they die. Being absent at that moment can leave a permanent scar.

Fortunately, it is becoming more and more accepted that this is the way the health services should develop for the dying, and in general. The services should give more support to people in their own homes and this means making specialist support mobile. Hospitals will continue to be needed for treatments which cannot be given elsewhere but they will be less the places for long stay. Economics alone should decide that, but with the ever-present danger in all fields that hospital services will be cut before proper community and home care has been built up.

But there is a new danger ahead. In the reformed National Health Service the emphasis is on primary care from GPs and district nurses and others – which is as it should be – but the need for specialists for terminally ill people is not being recognised in the right way. Hospice-type Home Care Teams are to have more and more of an advisory role as well as training and encouraging GPs and district nurses to raise the standards of the care they give to their patients. There is something to be said for this arrangement. The experience of the specialists can in that way be spread out over more patients. But the hands-on care and the 24-hour cover given to their patients by Home Care Teams should not be put in jeopardy, as it unfortunately now is. The Home Care nurses should continue to be involved in both hands-on care and in giving information direct to patients. GPs and district nurses cannot have the depth of experience that the St Joseph's nurses had. These nurses should be the model and not some different arrangement employed which owes far too much to the insistent (and for this purpose inappropriate) goal of cost effectiveness.

Older people

Up to this point we have been speaking as if all the patients had full-time, though untrained and unpaid, carers, when we know that is only true of a few. Some had only part-time, sometimes very part-time carers, and amongst these the most important distinction was of age. The few younger people were by and large the most unfortunate of all. They did not seem to have formed warm and enduring relationships which could be carried over into their adversity. Old angers and frustrations were still smouldering. Their marriages had failed, or were unsatisfactory, or had never existed, and, however dutiful their children, the relationship could hardly fail to be scarred by the past. This is not to say that a good death was unattainable, only that it was that much more difficult to achieve.

Older people are different. We mentioned them in Chapter 2 as mostly having had good deaths, fitting for their age. They were not amongst the fighters who held on with such admirable tenacity to the small pleasures of life, and the consolation of their own spirits. These were outstanding amongst the middle-aged. The older people were not fighters but accepters. They had got to the point where they would agree with the Chinese General who said that of the fifty-six possible courses of action on the battlefield, the best is usually to surrender, and, we would say, absorbed themselves in memories of the past. These can go back to childhood and great events like war which have figured large in their lives. Marshall has pointed out that many old people write the 'last chapter' of their lives through going back to earlier chapters, reviewing them and reaching the happy conclusion that their life had been pretty good.[8] Jack Dickson recollected the market.

> We all know how to tie up eight empty baskets. We all went into the competition for basket carrying, twelve on our heads, carrying a hundredweight of potatoes. It was a lovely life then.

Harold went back to his boyhood.

Sometimes we went tiddling on to Wanstead Flats. We'd take lard sandwiches and a bottle of cold tea and a jam jar and we'd sit and talk and eat . . . and we played football. We'd walk over to the Flats and play football there and we'd walk back. We'd be really tired by the time we got back. I've been going over in my mind the different way I used to lace my boots.

The behaviour of the older people can also be explained in terms of their social relationships, or rather the absence of them. People with full-time carers were surrounded by warmth and love which made their death both good and bad, good because they had so much support, bad because they had in consequence so much to lose, as did their survivors. But the older, without so many ties, had less to live for and less to lose, and, in a way, most to gain from death. Since the people they had been closest to in life were already dead, their own death would not generate further loss but might be the means of overcoming it. They might be (some thought they *would* be) re-united with the person they had been joined to before. The love which could tie some people to life could tie others to death. One death may well cause another; a death can also cancel another.

The wider community

The comparison made so far has been related to a central dilemma: the closer the web of human affection around the dying, from one point of view, the better; from another point of view, the worse. The dilemma has become all the sharper because the setting in which the drama takes place is so restricted, with so few actors to move around the dying and the death-bed. The relationships, where they exist at all, are intense and very private, without the softening, meliorating and transformative effect which a wider community can produce.

When considering what happens after as well as before, it becomes obvious that in summarising the enquiry it is not enough to compare one death with another within our tiny group – though we have done that too – but that, particularly when the bereaved are considered as well, for almost all there is something missing. They are almost all lacking another of the attributes of a good death – or a *better* death than almost any we have mentioned. They are almost all lacking, and we think wanting, the presence of a wider community, of people and of spiritual as well as material support. A hospice, even well-run hospice wards, as temporary communities can give something of this sense but they cannot be the same as more durable communities to which the dying and the bereaved can belong long before and long after the death.

Whether older or younger, the people we talked to were supported not just by home nurses but by advanced drugs and advanced technology. These are the achievement of thousands of dedicated research teams cooperating together in their own specialised community with their own private but universal languages which span the world. After all had been done that could be came an uneasy silence and an awkward shuffling. Before and at a death people might know more or less what to do.[9] Afterwards the support services fade away. The house of the dead looks the same as any other house, even if some of those who pass by now avert their eyes from it until the portents of something alarming have settled. The most tremendous and mysterious event can pass as though it is everyday, trivial, leaving each time a few survivors to find such solace as they can and deal as best they can, but in private, with their shock and their almost overwhelming grief. There is no match between the events which are happening inside, to the spectator within the breast, and the events outside, in a workaday world which with indecent haste resumes its customary routines.

But it is more difficult to endure for those who remain in the here and now. The bereaved should have support of a kind that includes the dying, the dead and the grieving. The four main needs are for

1 Making funerals more personal
2 Death to be prolonged beyond the funeral
3 Continuity to be established between the dead and the living
4 Death to regenerate morality and human solidarity.

In discussing them we shall go well beyond the bounds of our own enquiry but always with our informants very much in mind.

1 More personal funerals

We will start by describing an actual funeral of one of our patients, Kenneth again. It was a relatively traditional affair.

Kenneth had lived in the same place for the better part of his life, he was known by many local people, and the church he attended was hardly more than a stone's throw from his home. The news got round that he had died. As a result, people filled the back rows of the church. They joined 'the family' who took their place in the front, 70 to 100 relatives of Kenneth and his wife, all dressed in black from head to toe, each in their different relationship to the dead man, with the immediate family at the front and the others occupying pews at the right distance from the coffin, to sing the well-known hymns and watch the well-known priest go through the proceedings.

By present-day standards the show of solidarity was impressive and gave a measure of assurance that they were not alone to the principal mourners, who led the procession in and led the procession out on the way to the crematorium. The gathering gave to the bereaved and the children and grandchildren the sense that the death mattered to many more people than those in the immediate family.

But the funeral seemed to lose sight of the dead man, as though when he was shut into his coffin everything about him was shut down too. The only reference which brought Kenneth into the proceedings was when from the pulpit, in a kind of prose poem written by Canon Scott Holland in the last century and which has become immensely popular, inappropriate words were put into his mouth.

> Death is nothing at all. I have only slipped away into the next room. Call me by my old familiar name, speak to me in the easy way which you always used. Put no difference into your tone; wear no forced air of solemnity or sorrow. Laugh as we always laughed at the little jokes we enjoyed together. Play, smile, think of me, pray for me. Life means all that it ever meant. It is the same as it ever was; there is absolutely unbroken continuity. All is well.

The presumption of immortality was domesticated by the strange assertion that death had changed nothing, was nothing, as if after the cremation the funeral party could return home to find Kenneth waiting to greet them or, at any rate, to call to them from the next room in which he had died.

About the actual Kenneth and his actual life there was no word. So much was the priest absorbed in the grand story of the

Son of God and how he saved mankind from death that he had no time for God's particular creation whose death had brought them all together. The basic service from the 1662 Prayer Book does not have any place even for the name of the deceased. Dust can become dust, ashes ashes, without seeming to have taken the shape of a human being in the interim. Many priests and ministers still do not bother to find out anything about the dead person from family and friends, and fail to draw out their history, their characteristics and their achievements in their relationship to the collective history of which the dead have been part. Their failure leaves the congregation cold and uninvolved.

The mourners want to hear about the person they have lost, have praise for him or her, respond to an effort to bring him or her alive again at least in words, and, by implication anyway, be led in a lament for the departed. It is not just the fault of the clergy. Most of the crematoria in this country are run by local authorities who customarily allow only twenty minutes for the duty priest – or tame vicar as he is called – to gabble his way through the service before the next coffin is moved in. One change to present practice which would bring about a larger improvement than anything else would be to have the main service in a church or hall en route to the crematorium or cemetery.

A contrasting church

We came across another church in the inner city near our patch which was in sharp contrast. The minister, Rev. Jim Fallon, was one of the chaplains at St Joseph's Hospice. He came from the north of Scotland where many of the old death-traditions have survived, as they do, to a greater extent than in the cities, in the Celtic fringe generally and in rural areas of England. His early experience determined him to go back to his roots.

He had taken over a near derelict church building and, before too long, another near empty church which he hoped to bring back to life by the care he took to help people cope with death. Working in league with a local funeral director he, or after he had shown the way, one of the many assistants and counsellors whom he had recruited to the church from the bereaved, spent enough time with the family to get a real feel for the deceased. The assistant could stay to help in the home if necessary until the funeral was over. It was best of all if he, as the minister, met the deceased while they were still alive because then he could speak from some personal knowledge. At the funeral service he greeted the mourners when they arrived in the church before his carefully prepared eulogy, and left with them afterwards, putting his own cloak around the shoulders of the chief mourner if he thought it would be comforting. He visited the family again after the funeral.

Each part of the service was shaped to the particular needs of the person and the family. Much of it depended upon their ethnic group. His West Indian parishioners prefer open coffins and a fiery sermon and the nearest relatives heap the earth into the grave while gospel hymns are sung. This was fine with him, as were any other individual variations, particularly where people are traumatised by death because of previous family estrangements. A man of 52 who had a large family had for many years been estranged from them, from each of his ex-wives and his six legitimate and seven illegitimate children. He had been dead for three months before the police broke down the door of his flat. A son was called to arrange the funeral. Jim's task was to effect as much of a reconciliation as possible between the dead and the living, and to talk through some of the guilt and remorse, before he could get the wholehearted help of the children in going through with the funeral of their father. Death was a reconciliation.

Not only the chief mourner or mourners but anyone in the church was invited to come back to it again. And come they did, first for consolation themselves, for the personal support they got and for the ritual observances of the church, and, later, for the consolation they could bring to others who were dying or bereaved or just miserable. Deep feelings were recognised, encouraged and channelled.

When we first spoke with the minister, his church was full on Sundays, and the building not too far from full on weekdays, with a large nursery established on the premises for the children of the neighbourhood, and many other activities going on. An empty church had been taken over and filled. Death was the gateway to life.

Jim Fallon was a churchman who believed, in a literal sense, in the resurrection of Jesus Christ. But leave aside the literalness, and he is perfectly prepared to change the emphasis in the service if it is not in tune with what the deceased would have wanted, or what the mourners want. There are not all that many free-thinkers who would not acknowledge the value of what he and the members of his rapidly growing congregation attempt to do. They provided a stage on which emotions can be acted out, a common humanity celebrated and some prospect of consolation held forth.

A new practice

Partly because so many funeral services are so open to criticism, a new practice seems to be gathering some momentum. It gives (as in the Fallon church) much more prominence to what is often called the 'eulogy', meaning to speak well of the dead person's life. Bringing the dead person to life in this way will often be fully in accord (as we have seen) with the feelings of those who are suffering most. For the point is to describe the person as the people around him or her saw him or her, with quirks and faults as well as virtues – the rounded humanity – brought out. The address can be given by a member of the family, or someone they choose who knew the deceased, or it can be a priest, or, for non-religious funerals, a fellow-humanist who feels confident to speak on behalf of others. Where this approach is followed, the priest, or the equivalent in secular funerals who does the formal speaking, can do this adequately only if they take the trouble to visit the family before the funeral and get as complete a picture as possible of the dead person.

Even more striking about the Fallon church were the lengths to which he and his people were prepared to go to extend sup-port to the bereaved well beyond the funeral. They demonstrated how valuable the bereaved can be (to themselves as well as others) once they are able to bring some comfort to people who have gone through the same terrible experience as themselves.

There has been the same tendency in other countries, with a new role of 'celebrant', as described by Walter,[10] appearing in Australia, New Zealand and, to a lesser extent, in Holland. In Australia the new movement grew out of the office of marriage celebrant which was instituted in the 1970s when the people who acted for marriages were asked to lead funerals as well. There are also specialised funeral celebrants who can be either priests or laypeople. The common characteristic, whether they draw on religious or secular philosophy, is that they focus 'on the life, character and relationships of the one who has died'.[11] Humanists can take to the practice more readily because, without a time-hallowed service to fall back on, they have had to make more of the deceased. But more priests appear to be moving in the same direction. The authors of this book, in conjunction with other colleagues, have attempted to give the movement a further impetus by starting a National Funerals College.[12]

2   Prolong support beyond the grave

The second need foreshadowed by the second church goes well beyond the funeral, as well as including it, and puts a stop to any notion that the death can be sealed off after the burial or crema-tion. For the mourners, the funeral is a support as well as an ordeal. They can be caught up in an occasion which, in a small but significant way, demonstrates the benefit of community back-ing. But for them it can be the prelude to a period of melancholy which is all the more of a trial because it can be so intensely private at a time when privacy is not what is needed, or not only what is needed.

We should at this point go back to the people described in the last chapter who could not accept that their dead were dead. They did not wake up one morning and say to themselves – 'I want him or her back, I am bringing him back' – as though they could do what no doctor can do and raise people from the dead as effortlessly as if they were being woken up from sleep. It just happened involuntarily, whether they wanted it to or not. Harold was there lying in the bed next to you, Donald was waiting for you when you got back from your shopping, the dead Derek was a presence who filled your flat. It could be alarming. It could even make people fear they were going mad. But the comfort of it far outdid the alarm. If a ghost, the ghost was 'there', and it (he?, she?) was on the whole friendly, even though so little like ordinary humdrum life. The ghost was in some ways more real than ordinary life.

The people who held these views are by no means alone. According to a general survey covering the country as a whole, and some other countries as well, the dying and the bereaved in our sample are in the company of a majority of the population. The British Social Attitudes Survey which is conducted regularly

reports answers to some questions about religion.[13] They are given
in Table 1.

Table 1 Religious beliefs and observances, per cent

	Britain	USA	Republic of Ireland	Northern Ireland
Belief in God	69	94	95	95
That God is concerned personally with people	37	77	77	80
Life after death	55	78	80	78
Heaven	54	86	87	90
Religious miracles	45	73	73	77
Hell	28	71	53	74
The devil	28	47	49	69
Belief in the Bible as the actual or the inspired word of God	44	83	78	81
Affiliated with a denomination	64	93	98	92
Attend service two or three times monthly	16	43	78	58
Have had intense religious experience	28	33	22	24

Number of informants: 1,221

Even though religious belief is on this score less in Britain than
in the USA and Ireland, it is still striking that 69 per cent of
British people express a belief in God, 64 per cent consider
themselves affiliated to a church and 55 per cent believe in life
after death. There are higher proportions amongst older people.
If the questions were understood in the same way, there has even
been an increase in the proportion believing in an afterlife.
Gorer's 1964 figure was 49 per cent.[14]

So the belief in an afterlife is certainly not confined to a few,
perhaps unusual, people in East London nor to people who have
suffered a bereavement. Nor can the experience be dismissed as
a mere passing hallucination of no particular significance. For it
is as common as it is profound. It has been reported before, in
industrialised countries, and, much more widely, in many other
societies besides ours and in the religions of many other societies,
and of many ethnic minorities now represented in Britain. The
conventional modern view of death is that it occurs in an instant:

that instant when clinical death gives way to brain death, and the person who up to that second has been alive is suddenly alive no more. A well-oiled hinge turns the living present instantaneously into the dead past. The sociological view, reflecting the multifold experience of mourners as social beings, is that not only dying but death also is a lengthy business. We have attempted to do something to relieve cancer of its bad reputation by acknowledging there is some virtue in a long-drawn-out illness, and now we are saying that there is virtue, too, in a death which is prolonged beyond the grave. We are all of us soon to become the past but it does not have to be instantaneous, as if one day we are flesh and blood and the next day marble.

The bereaved whom we saw were recovering their dead and holding on to them, not so much because they wanted to as because they had to. The *Rubaiyat* was only partly right when it said that nobody has experienced death, or Wittgenstein when he said that 'Death is not an event in life, it is not lived through.'[15] The still living live through it and yet stay with it. People knew at one level of their minds that the dead were dead, but they could not accommodate that realisation without also harbouring an image of the dead as not being dead. The dead were dead and not-dead. The constant contrast between the dead and the non-dead was what made the comfort also so tragic. This was especially so when the bereaved were reminded of their loss by anything which recalled the dead – an old letter, a coat still hanging up in the hall, or suddenly wondering 'what would he have thought of that?', and asking him[16] – and by the recurrence of significant dates.

Why should the day when the person died matter each time it came around, and even more so when it was the anniversary of the death? It was as if there was a kind of numerological magic at work which both allowed people to prepare for the feelings that could be aroused by the recurrence of the regular cycles (and so to some extent control them) and to be almost bowled over by the onrush when the day came. The deathday succeeded the birthday (though the birthdays of the dead person were not forgotten either, and their symbolic celebration of life). Just as, in a symbolic sense, people are born again on a birthday, so do people die again on a series of deathdays. The first annual deathday could be a bit of both, the day on which the dead die again, but with less pain to the bereaved than before, and for that reason also, the day on which the bereaved could take further their return to ordinary life. Whether or not there is some sign of a rebirth happening then, it is only after the lapse of a period of time that people can begin to feel that they are 'letting go', this being a common phrase for the new profession of bereavement counselling. It is only after the necessary 'grief work' has been done that the bereaved can let go of the dead person and return, 'reborn', to ordinary life; and it may be that only if people are able to do that, will they, when their time comes, be able to say, like Tennyson:

Let me go: take back thy gift.[17]

But 'letting go' does not need to be complete, and it would be false to suggest that 'letting go' could, or should, ever be anything more than a state which coincides with the continued life of the dead.

In the most technological of societies people are going through this primordial experience in their millions as countless millions more have gone through it since time immemorial, millions of years ago at the birth of the human race. Mumford points out that amongst palaeolithic men the dead were the first to have a permanent dwelling, a cavern, a mound, a collective barrow.

Soon after one picks up man's trail in the earliest campfire or chipped-stone tool one finds evidence of interests and anxieties that have no animal counterpart; in particular, a ceremonious concern for the dead, manifested in their deliberate burial – with growing evidence of pious apprehension and dread.[18]

The crucial difference now is that the experience is not recognised, not supported and not harnessed effectively to any sort of renewal of society by a supporting body of ritual and observance. In this distancing from notions of the afterlife and by the threadbareness of the ritual with which it surrounds death, modern society is very much the exception amongst the general run of societies, historically and even contemporaneously.

In other societies less touched by our passion for novelty, and more attuned to the traditional, death has been allowed its own substantial duration. Robert Hertz, a pupil of Émile Durkheim, gave the first systematic account of the 'double obsequies' which are widespread in so many different places. This is one of the keys to the long-drawn-out ritual which death can give rise to when it is *not* regarded as instantaneous. He said that the ritual 'implies the passage from one group to another: an exclusion, i.e. a death, and a new integration, i.e. a rebirth'.[19] Such a passage has to be slow because there is so much to be forgotten and learnt, and so many painful adjustments to be made in behaviour as the emphasis shifts away from death and over to birth, but with the two being indissolubly linked.

In Western society a variant of the long Hertzian death has been preserved in orthodox Jewish practice. There is the Shiva ceremony which continues for seven days after the funeral, with friends and relatives coming together to be with the mourners, and with evening prayers every night in the home; the *Sheloshim* according to which there is abstinence for thirty days; *Kaddish*, the mourning prayer which is recited every day in the synagogue by the chief male mourner not for a year but, in accord with a lunar calendar, for eleven months; and the second service at the end of that period when the gravestone is dedicated. The pattern goes from the most severe grief to more formal observance.[20] Also notable are the Jewish Burial Societies (and the Muslim for that matter) which provide a comprehensive service for their members, all the way from the care of the body to the care of the soul. The traditional mourner's food – things like lentils, bagels, hard-boiled eggs – symbolise the roundness and continuity of life.

In the middle ages the existence of purgatory served something of the same purpose. There people would wait to be purified enough to go on to heaven or, if they did not qualify, to the other place. The survivors could greatly affect the outcome, and protect themselves from evil spirits not yet put to rest, by the strenuousness of their prayers for the dead. A kind of democracy ruled over purgatory and one (as in many democracies) that lent itself to corrupt practice, in this case by the church – this being one of the causes of the Reformation. But the notion of purgatory would not have lasted so long (and still survive in popular speech) had it not been in tune with the grief of the mourners, unless it offered them some 'work' that they could do to influence what happened to the dead and unless the period of waiting had its term, most aptly a year. With the ceremonial that marked the end of it, the soul could be released for its further journey and the bereaved released to throw off the last of their mourning clothes and rejoin ordinary life.

Of all this, there are many practices remaining in the church. The Roman Catholic Church makes much of requiem masses, said on the anniversary of the death or birthday or wedding day. All Souls Day (2 November) is an occasion for all the dead to be remembered. In the Church of England Eucharist services on the anniversary are the equivalent of requiem masses, and since 1928 when the day was restored, there can be a memorial Eucharist on All Souls Day. The Free Churches do not have the same tradition of praying for the departed, although many chapels have Books of Remembrance and the names of the dead are mentioned in Sunday services. But many people are left out of these observances.

Whether with or without the aid of purgatory and some transitional stage between life and death, Christianity has in its central myth drawn out the death, and the birth, and the rebirth, into a year-long series of archetypal events. They are tied into the life cycle which all nature goes through in the course of a solar year. Following the calendar of the seasons is a clue to the success of the church (which it shares with other world religions) in having brought together so many billions of individual people into membership and also spread its calendar so wide.

Nothing is so beautiful as Spring –
When weeds, in wheels, shoot long and lovely and lush;
Thrush's eggs look little low heavens, and thrush
Through the echoing timber does so rinse and wring
The ear, it strikes like lightnings to hear him sing;[21]

Spring, as celebrated by Gerard Manley Hopkins, and particularly at Easter, is when the crucifixion, the rebirth – the resurrection – and the conception are all celebrated. On 25 March at the time of the Feast of the Annunciation, the good news of the coming birth given to the Virgin Mary by the Archangel Gabriel is celebrated. This is nine months before the birth itself and just before the new year is born; and in between and in the three months after the birth, the life of Christ, and in symbolic form the life of everyone, is commemorated by the appropriate ritual and its accompanying poetry and music.

If there is to be any large revival of ritual around death,[22] it will, in an ecological age, need to echo the cycle of birth and death – the death and the birth – of all natural things; and it will also need to relate the individual to the whole more convincingly than it does now. It is all very well summarising life and death into a year, and marvellous to draw the comparison with that part of nature which dies and is reborn within a year. But the bereaved also need rituals that are more particular to them. These are the markers for remembrance in every church – the prayers for the dead, All Souls Day, the other services.

People who belong to a church may be able to match up the stages through which they pass in their individual bereavement with observances which give them some public support for what they are going through. That in itself may be some comfort to them, as it can be just to be together with people suffering in the same way as themselves. Whether or not they are active members of a church, they are liable to be lonely in their loss. This matters to the dying as well as to the survivors. If both mourners and their relatives, friends and acquaintances, had known what to do on the occasion of a death, or deaths, the dying would have known what was to happen after death because he or she would have been through it before when other people died.

If support from the community ceases with the funeral (unsatisfactory as the funeral often is) support can, therefore, cease when it is most needed. People make their own adjustments (as we have seen in the last chapter) by believing in an afterlife, and should not be thought of as in any way strange for doing so. But not many can manage all by themselves. Carers need care as much as the dying, after as well as before the death. We don't expect a great revival of the custom of the double obsequies under that or any other name. But at least it needs to be recognised that something equivalent to, as well as different from, the Home Care team is needed for the bereaved. Such teams could be based on churches, as they were in the Fallon church, or they could grow out of the bereavement and befriending services which already exist. They are themselves a recent and welcome phenomenon, and need every encouragement they can get. Some of the organisations which are looking out for volunteers figure in Appendix III.

3   Establish continuity between the dead and the living

Some people consider it obvious that death is 'the end', and that any belief to the contrary is no more than wishful, weak-minded fantasy. They can even take pride in their realism and face up to death with as much composure as those who believe in something after death. But one has to ask the realists what they mean by 'the end'. The end of what? Of their own individual lives, yes. But of life, no. Life goes on, and goes on because they have themselves shaped the way it goes on. 'Harold's alive,' said Lilian, 'as long as the children are alive. There's so much of him in them.' Or, she could have said, his grandchildren and great grand-children, in reducing proportions but ad infinitum. All parents can say the same.

Of course, from one point of view these are platitudes. But they are platitudes with an edge to them for they allow those who accept that death is an end for them as individuals to recog-nise that their end is not the end of all. They may not be able to believe (as some but not all of our informants did) in individual immortality. But they can believe in, and even find some comfort in, collective immortality. Julia Searle did not think that 'she' and her own sense of herself as the unique Julia was going in some way to survive after her death. But she could think, even though she had no children to carry on many of her characteristics, that something of her was going to survive, through Maria and her other friends.

The commonsense experience of parents and others who are not has been paralleled by one of the great scientific achievements of this century. The geneticists and molecular biologists have shown that continuities are much more literal than anyone would have thought. Like souls which have in some religions also been thought of as migrating from one body to another, the physical migrants are the genes which control so many of life's manifes-tations in every one of the thousand million million cells making up an average human body, and their patterned interaction. The genes at least do not die but persist as they are transported from one body to another and combine and re-combine in order to make and sustain another body which is different. In the words of Richard Dawkins:

> The genes are the immortals, or rather, they are defined as genetic entities that come close to deserving the title. We, the individual survival machines in the world, can expect to live a few more decades. But the genes in the world have an

expectation of life that must be measured not in decades but in thousands and millions of years. . . .

Genes, like diamonds, are forever, but not quite in the same way as diamonds. It is an individual diamond crystal that lasts, as an unaltered pattern of atoms. DNA molecules don't have that kind of permanence. The life of any one physical DNA molecule is quite short – perhaps a matter of months, certainly not more than one lifetime. But a DNA molecule could theoretically live on in the form of *copies* of itself for a hundred million years.[23]

We are not saying that the remarkable durability of DNA and RNA in our bodies should make any 'survival machine' jump for joy on the grounds that, because some tiny but elemental part of us which is in every one of our multitudinous cells can defy death, 'we' can; but it does demonstrate that though we die, not the whole of us does.

It is much the same with societies which are also reproduced because people copy (and miscopy) each other. A central concern of sociology is with the processes whereby all societies maintain themselves, while also changing and adapting in order to do so, and succeed in this while the composition of their membership is constantly turning over as some people give up membership and others enter upon it. This is most obvious with great innovators whose influence can be felt hundreds or thousands of years after they have lived. 'Blow on a dead man's embers and, like the rubbing of an old lamp in a fairy story, a miracle may take place.'[24] But everyone takes part in handing on the culture, not just the new bits of it and the parts that do not change, and which embody the experience of many generations. This accumulated experience matters more than any current innovation. We would say that everyone's influence will be felt for 'ever'. It is inconceivable to us that the undertakings of a person, the children he or she has, how he or she approaches death, what he or she says that appears trivial at the time, will be completely extinguished. It will all bounce about in the future. We know that such an unattributable future, with no name tags on it, will not satisfy by any means all the seekers. No matter: nothing will.

We ourselves are grandchildren and greatgrandchildren and members of societies with a continuity to them. The air around us is filled with communications from the dead, from Jesus and

Buddha, from Shakespeare and Napoleon. More and more of the past is being thrust into the present. A series of prosthetic devices which started with the writing down of speech and the painting of pictures, and has continued with the modern media, has produced a collective memory which is reproducing and misreproducing the past on a scale boggling in its detail. The present is being crammed with the past – although not in the way that ritual encapsulated tradition. As revivals, the 1940s, 1950s, 1960s, 1970s and 1980s can all be playing simultaneously in the 1990s – like an undressing in a striptease which continues in slow motion for half a century.

We are the children, and we are the parents, and we will be embodied in the ongoing continuity just as we embody what has happened before us. What we have is most definitely an afterlife. But the afterlife is not the afterlife of an individual alive now, but an afterlife in others who are in the same flow, linked by being made up of some of the same atoms, some of the same genes, some of the same morality, some of the same habits, some of the same ideas, some of the same primordial fears and hopes, as we who are going to die before them.

But, perhaps in part because there is no mystery about collective immortality, by no means everyone can find enough solace in it to make their minds tranquil when they are getting ready for the final merging of their personal individuality into the impersonal collectivity. Indeed, for some there is no solace at all; the reaction can be precisely the other way round: a mixture of indignation and grief. The cruellest thing about a death lies precisely in that collective continuity. Life goes on without the dead (and it wrongly appears) just as if they had never existed. The buses rush to their stops but with quite different people looking out of the windows. The planes take off for New York but with only strangers in them. The choir picks up the haunting melody and she or he is not there to hear it.

Many of our informants were like that. Whatever they experienced, something was lacking from it – the presence of the person who was no longer their flesh-and-blood companion. The collective immortality, if they thought about it at all, was much too impersonal for them to draw any solace from. They wanted something much more personal and specific to them and found it in a belief in the afterlife of the person to whom they had been so close. Their experience raises the question whether the individual loss can be made a little less searing if it is directly related to the overall continuity. This brings us on to the last section of the chapter.

4   Death to regenerate morality[25]

There can be no gilding over of the finitude. It represents the utmost loss, and one which can only seem to have some point to it if the loss is offset by some gain. There needs to be a moral purpose, which death can serve, and a purpose which can have a general bearing on the lives of ordinary people in ordinary times, not just in wartime when people sacrifice themselves almost gladly for their country or their group and to some degree do it voluntarily, not involuntarily.

On morality David Hume is as good a guide as any, and a better guide than most. He asked, on what foundation is any system of ethics to rest? It can only rest on a view of human nature. Human beings, he said, come into the world endowed by their human constitution with the strong sentiment of self-love and the weak sentiment of benevolence. Benevolence was his word for fellow-feeling, and fellow-feeling was the father of all morality.

> While the human heart is compounded of the same elements as at present, it will never be wholly indifferent to public good, nor entirely unaffected with the tendency of characters and manners. And though this affection of humanity may not generally be esteemed so strong as vanity and ambition, yet being common to all men, it can alone be the foundation of morals, or of any general system of blame or praise.[26]

It is fellow-feeling, for fellows they have never met and never will, which stirs people when there is a catastrophe in Africa or Asia.

What have these axioms of Hume got to do with death? To make the link it is necessary to add to his another statement of our own with at least a pretension to being an axiom: Death, being also common to all men, is the ever-available assistant to fellow feeling. We are not saying that death is always thus, any more (we think) than Hume would have denied that some people are so evil that to search inside their minds for the spark of benevolence would be a wishful fancy. Death can lay waste individual hearts, even whole countries, and may yet lay waste the whole world through nuclear disaster, with no redeeming consequence. Death can live up to its common reputation, especially when brought on with foul intent. Make-believe death can also be used to feed every sort of imagining, including the most sinister and destructive.

The person at home in the middle of an array of knobs and buttons which control his immediate environment can, with the aid of other robots, summon up at will the most amazing fantasies. An immense fairy-story world[27] is ready to feed the illusion, for adults as well as children, that no-one needs to die. Artists contribute to this illusion, as they have always done, by imagining how to control time, make it stand still, leap forward or turn back, and their reach has been greatly enlarged by the media. The festival of death and of horror associated with it has become one of our favourite modern games. No Nero or Caligula was served by as many gladiators as a single child in any industrialised country. It has been calculated that by the time an average US child has reached the age of 14 he or she could be expected to have seen 18,000 people killed on TV[28] and, we are sure, to have seen hosts of immortals – as they are called – who are sufficiently immune from death to come through alive. When all their enemies are slaughtered they reappear again and again in other equally horrific dramas, and keep reappearing on the screen even after they are long reported dead.

But we are arguing that actual death is not like these fantasy deaths. There can always, or nearly always, be a counter-tendency, a constructive tendency, a thrust towards regeneration which can be used to compensate or go some way towards compensating, for the loss.[29] Germany was not buried in Auschwitz. This is partly because death casts its own special light on the self-love which Hume counted the strongest sentiment in the human heart. Only saints can extinguish it completely. Even as they approach death, many people are still keen to enhance their reputation and earn admiration for their fortitude, love for their demonstration of love, or gratitude for their display of gratitude. But for most ordinary people, unsaintly but not totally self-centred, the approach of death, or the contemplation of it after it has occurred, does at least raise the great question about where self-love has got them.

What profiteth it them? The question has been asked of people so often because it is a question which most people can hardly avoid asking themselves. Where has their self-love brought them? It has brought some people the accumulation of possessions which they have been conditioned to think of as extensions of themselves. But the material goods which in our society bulk so large in our value systems do not stand them in good stead in their final crisis. Most of the manifestations and fruits of self-regard cannot stand up to the harsh scrutiny of death. 'We brought nothing into this world, and it is certain we can carry nothing out' (Timothy 1: 6).

Hence the attempt of many people near death – and not only those afraid of hell-fire – to make amends for some of the damage they have done in their lifetimes. One of the offices performed by religions was to provide means by which, before it was too late, repentance could be expressed and good deeds performed – sometimes less for the general good than for the good of the church which had arrogated to itself such influence with the other side. That kind of rush to morality is much less evident than it used to be, partly because the church has had to surrender some of its power. But the general tendency has not been much diminished, nor its beneficent effect.

As the strong sentiment becomes weaker, the weak sentiment gets stronger. If self-love becomes more pointless when there will soon be no self to love, what is there left but fellow-feeling? When all else is stripped away, what remains is a vulnerable human being who can yet be strengthened, even to some extent reconciled, by the most fundamental of feelings, the feelings of common humanity, and who arouses those same feelings in others.

If that is how it often is with the dying, before they withdraw into themselves, it can also be the same, if to a lesser extent, for the carers and even for the bystanders. Altruism of different degrees can be as contagious as hatred or malice. This is because, more than any other condition of humankind, except perhaps birth, the death of another makes you think of your own death. Even if you do not cross yourself – to ward off evil or to express sympathy – you may feel like doing something of the sort. Primitive superstitions can be aroused, as can premonitions as well as sympathies, despite all the efforts that will be made by doctors and funeral directors to conceal the corpse which will one day be yours. You don't need to be told for whom the bell tolls or from whence comes the smoke puffing out of the crematorium chimney.

Death is *the* common experience which can make all members of the human race feel their common bonds and their common humanity. The presence of death, for all its terror and bitterness (as the rabbit is snared or the fish hooked), can generate the mystical sense of unity with other people which transcends the boundaries of the body and the self. In the words of the metaphysical poet Traherne:[30]

Then was my Soul my only All to me,
A living endless eye,
Just bounded with the sky
Whose power, whose act, whose essence, was to see.

It is what Freud called the 'oceanic feeling', the 'sensation of eternity', the sense of 'something limitless, unbounded' or the sense of 'oneness with the universe'.[31] It is like the experience of At-One-Ment which figures in Jewish religion and which finds a different expression in the many near-death experiences which have now been recorded.[32] The experience is linked to a sense of the reality of the unseen.

It is as if there were in the human consciousness a *sense of reality, a feeling of objective presence, a perception* of what we may call *'something there'*, more deep and more general than any of the special and particular 'senses' by which the current psychology supposes existent realities to be originally revealed.[33]

Our carers were not exerting themselves for the sake of any personal gain. They exerted themselves the more, and endured the more, because death was in the offing and maybe, in an expression of genuine altruism, because they could get no recompense from the dying person in exchange for what they were doing for him or for her. Reversing the usual order of things, the less the reward, the more the effort – thus, when near the sacred, reversing the common-or-garden behaviour of the ordinary profane world. Nor were they wracked with grief because they were going to gain anything from it. On the contrary, they were for a time to lose sleep, lose their zest for life, lose the meaning that their lives had until they were plunged into this misery. They were mourning the others who had departed earlier – their mothers and fathers, their grandmothers and grandfathers – and those in the future (including themselves) who were soon going to depart on the same journey.

But perhaps even better witnesses were the people who possessed none of the obligation which kinship demands. They were not acting out of conventional duty. We are thinking of the people from the community, as distinct from close family relatives, of the kind mentioned in Chapter 4, who came to Donald's funeral – of the members of the British Legion, for instance, who were so well represented in the church. We are thinking of a spontaneous demonstration before Julia's funeral when neighbours arranged flowers outside and below her window. 'When I looked out from my window', said Maria, 'the flowers circled the tree in a great big heart shape. It was lovely.' We are thinking of the neighbours who unobtrusively, and without even being asked, acted like kin when they were not – as one Mary who might have been named Martha came downstairs to bring Arthur, on his own in his flat, a nightly drink of hot blackcurrant; or another Martha cooked a dinner for the even more lonely Dermot. The most telling of all, with almost symbolic overtones to it, was the incident related by Lilian Allen, when she was stopped in the street by strangers who lived near her but who had never spoken to her before. They said they had heard about the death of her husband. They said how sorry they were, and quietly listened to an account of all that had happened to her. No sympathy from anyone else was as warming as that.

The perpetual fund of goodwill which death can generate is there, has always been there and will always be there as long as humankind survives. The failing of the collective arrangements we now make is that we draw so parsimoniously on the fund and fail so often to top it up. It is a general failing, and therefore a failing of almost all the churches. Churchpeople almost seem to have forgotten that, by supporting the dead, they support the living; that ritual is a method of demonstrating fellow-feeling; that the structure of morality is in good part spun out from the vigour it can get from death. If it had not been for that compensation, and the expression it found in religion, death could have been too deadly to allow a general survival. The multiplication of death that any death can set off has to be held in check.

Students of society would say that the sense of unity is latent in all people and, without that, societies would be a great deal more fragile. Underlying all the stronger forces which keep

societies in being – the common traditions, the common languages, the common interests, the hierarchies of power – is a
weaker but universal force of gravity, of social gravity, which is
always acting to hold people together. It is like the physical force
of gravity, the ever-present force which holds the physical universe together, from our earth and the moon and the sun to the
furthest star in the furthest galaxy, and exists alongside other
forces, the electro-magnetic and the nuclear. Science has not yet
understood the physical force of gravity – why one mass is
attracted to another without any identifiable force acting between
them. Social science has not yet fully understood how the social
force of gravity operates either. But its manifestations can be
recognised in the tendency for people to identify with others, and
to have fellow-feeling for others as human beings, or, beyond
that, with all living flora or fauna. The force is particularly evident
at the time of death, or danger of death, when there can be a
kind of bonding together of the dead and the survivors. It is
notable that, insofar as there is such a force, it can draw people
not only to others who are still alive but to others who have died
before, and not only to those within the close family but to
other members of the human family, Jesus Christ or Buddha, the
Unknown Warrior or, less specifically, in their billions the great
hosts of the dead.

With such a possibility accessible to anyone it is easy enough
to recognise the value of the ritual which in many other societies
does, and in our society could, accompany the transition from
the first death to the second, and to rebirth. It does justice to the
sacrifice which death entails, and it invites people to identify
themselves with the ongoing community which is renewed by
death. The advantages of symbolising this tremendous transition
in a myth of a once human being, and His death and rebirth, is
obvious enough, especially when the story conjures up the hosts
who have been caught up in the same story before, sorrowed and
perhaps found some comfort in the externalisation and sharing
of that which is so painful.

Actors without lines

Some of those who cannot 'believe' in that story – though they
cannot, while human, be non-believers in the human story – can
perhaps admit that without the ritual the public acknowledgement

of a death can be a meagre affair which touches no more than the outer surface of a person. The same can easily happen to religous observance, indeed this can be even more hollow when the traditional is followed without anyone understanding what it portends.

If we are right in what we have said about the role of medicine in encouraging lingering illness, it has done something which will increasingly call into question the individualism which has made such a powerful alliance with technology. To some extent the focus could return to death and, if it does, we are bound to look again at the practices with which we surround it. Leaving aside the minorities with more well-entrenched traditions, at most contemporary deaths the mourners and others are actors without any lines, participants in a drama without parts to play. They can be hollow people, and if they begin more and more to feel there is a void, in time it will be filled, even perhaps with the churches in the lead, but with many affinities with people who belong to none. The traditional traditional may be terminal; but the new traditional, incorporating some of the old traditional but renewing it, and extending it even for a good period after death, may offer better prospects. Whether it will do so depends as much on life as on death – in other words on the general course taken by the great society – and, particularly, on whether the moral economy of that society is going to be visited with more of Hume's benevolence or the human sympathy of Adam Smith.

If the essential link between death and birth, and the way the linear spirals into the cyclical, is acknowledged, within the domain sketched out by this study the search could be on for new kinds of observance which could be relevant to the world which the movers of science and technology have built. This would involve taking death out of the closet and casket, into the open, and dealing with the fear of it by other means than courage, or at least not by that alone. What was most majestic about the death of Christ, or Socrates, or Hume, or many others, was their acceptance of death, and, though they had extraordinary courage, they had more than that. It is not by courage alone that the dead will be saved. Comical as well as serious though we all are, a belief which links death to life is also needed if, in society too, a great positive is to continue to come out of a great negative. The belief needs to be authentic as well as contemporary if it is to crystallise as well as strengthen a new view of the bonds between us which make us human, which make us into life.

Life lives on.
It is the lives, the lives, the lives, that die.[34]

Appendix I
List of patients

The first summary descriptions of the patients were given in Chapter 2. The page numbers on which these summaries were given are listed below. This is for the sake of readers who want to refer back from later in the book and to check on who was who.

Harold Allen	(page 18)
Dora Anstey	(page 13)
Jennifer Barnes	(page 16)
Walter Bliss	(page 23)
Kenneth Chandler	(page 17)
Alice Colyer	(page 25)
Jack Dickson	(page 24)
Dermot Donoghue	(page 11)
Arthur Jacobs	(page 26)
Donald Knight	(page 26)
Janet Rahman	(page 29)
Julia Searle	(page 32)
Carol Taylor	(page 18)
Derek Wood	(page 28)

Appendix II
Hospices, Macmillan nurses and other services

Hospices

Hospice care has developed over the same period of time as the Cancer Relief Macmillan Fund has developed its care units and nursing services. Much hospice development has taken place since the late 1960s but the origins go much further back than that.

> At the beginning of the 19th century, Mary Aikenhead, a lady of remarkable holiness and vision, devoted her life to the abandoned poor.... In 1815 she founded the religious order of the Sisters of Charity. Their first base was a small orphanage in Dublin.... In the year 1900 they came to England [responding]... to Cardinal Vaughan's expressed concern for the plight of the sick in the slums of London. Benefactors provided the sisters with a small house in Mare Street from which they could walk to the homes of the bedridden.... As soon as the adjacent house became available they combined and modified both to provide wards. The first patient, a 47 year old Hackney Tram Driver dying of consumption, was carried in by his friends on January 14th 1905.[1]

It was in St Josephs in the 1950s that Dame Cicely Saunders, as a medical officer, was able to develop techniques of pain control which she had earlier observed while working as a volunteer nurse in St Luke's Hospital.[2] The growth of the modern hospice movement can be traced back to Dr Saunders' opening in 1967 of St Christopher's Hospice, Sydenham, which has since become a model for similar institutions and a centre for teaching and research. St Christopher's inaugurated home care two years later, in 1969. The St Joseph's Hospice Home Care service was set up by Dr Richard Lamerton in 1975; he 'had seen a particular need to supplement the care of the Primary Health Care Teams in East London with their terminally ill patients'.[3] Beginning with a few charitable hospices in the 1960s, there were in 1994 133 independent or voluntary hospice units.

Although Hospice Care is principally for patients with advanced cancer many services (65 per cent of in-patient units) will consider applications from patients with other terminal illness.[4]

Palliative care

The innovative work of hospices has set the standard for achievement in good palliative care. Hospice care is not just for dealing with pain relief but goes beyond symptom control, attending to a patient's social, emotional and spiritual needs, as well as offering support to families. Since 1987 palliative medicine has been recognised as a speciality in its own right; this is largely the result of the pioneering work of hospices.

Palliative care is now a distinct medical speciality in the United Kingdom. It focuses on controlling pain and other symptoms, easing suffering and enhancing the life that remains. It integrates the psychological and spiritual aspects of care, to enable patients to live out their lives with dignity, as well as offering support to families both during the patient's illness and their bereavement. It offers a unique combination of care in hospices and at home.[5]

Macmillan nurses

From the turn of the century the Cancer Relief Macmillan Fund, founded in 1911 by Douglas Macmillan as the National Society for Cancer Relief, has spread information on the prevention and relief of cancer. Douglas Macmillan wanted

to see homes for cancer patients throughout the land, where attention will be provided freely or at low cost, as circumstances dictate . . . [and] . . . panels of voluntary nurses who can be detailed off to attend to necessitous patients in their own homes.[6]

By 1933 the Society was providing some families with grants for the cost of medicines, dressings and food and had appointed two full-time nurse visitors, in London and York. By 1975, Cancer Relief had built and equipped the first of its own cancer care units and now twelve such units stand in the grounds of NHS hospitals. Also in 1975 the Fund gave money for its first Macmillan nurse teams to care for patients in their own homes, with grants for this purpose made to St Joseph's Hospice in Hackney, whose staff were already visiting patients at home, St Colombia's Hospice in Edinburgh, and The Dorothy House Foundation in Bath. A DHSS report[7] in 1980 advised that future developments in terminal care should give priority to expanding home-care services.

The Cancer Relief Macmillan Fund responded with a large investment in the form of three-year grants to establish Macmillan nursing posts nationwide. Macmillan nurses are Registered General Nurses specially trained in pain and symptom control for cancer care and in giving emotional support to patients and their carers. As with the cancer care units, these nursing posts were funded for the first three years by Cancer Relief,[8] after which time full responsibility for them was taken over by the health authorities. There are now nearly a thousand such Macmillan nurses working closely with doctors, district nurses and health visitors, mostly in the community, caring for patients at home; some are attached to hospitals. They sometimes work individually and sometimes as part of a home care team or a hospital team. A large number of home care teams started by the Cancer Relief Macmillan Fund took the name 'Macmillan Nursing Service'[9] and although many such services are now independent of CRMF funding the name Macmillan has sometimes remained.[10]

Types of hospice care

Palliative care can be more or less interventionist depending on the setting and the approach of the care unit concerned.

> In the hospice setting, 'palliative' refers to the control of symptoms by the use of medications and non-pharmacological interventions. . . . This meaning is closest to the latin root 'pallium' – a cloak (OED). Oncologists use the term 'palliative' to refer to treatment which slows down or shrinks the cancer

at one or more sites for as long as possible, with no expectation of cure.[11]

Over the last twenty years, a large expansion in the number of hospice units has seen the emergence of many different palliative care units. They differ not only in size, location and source of funding but also in the way they embrace the hospice approach to care, that is the extent to which they use medical therapies, the nature of their psychosocial care, the extent of a family's involvement with the patient's care and the patterns of staff relations.[12] But hospice-type care has taken certain principal forms.

The first of these and the most familiar are the independent in-patient units with beds for terminally ill people such as St Christopher's and St Joseph's Hospices. In addition to the 133 such units, there are a further eleven Marie Curie Cancer Care Centres[13] and nine Sue Ryder Homes.[14] To these must be added the fifty continuing care units (from 1973 onwards) which represent hospice practice in a hospital setting. They are usually located in the grounds of an NHS hospital and offer in-patient care. Several were initially funded in whole or in part by the Cancer Relief Macmillan Fund. They are now funded and run by the NHS.

The second kind of service is represented by the home care service teams which may or may not be attached to a residential unit like St Joseph's Hospice. A home care team may consist of anything from a Macmillan nurse working alone to a team consisting of a doctor and Macmillan nurses and perhaps a social worker and even a chaplain. This 'team' offers advice and sometimes complementary help to the primary care team of GP, practice nurse and district nurse who give hands-on-care to patients at home. There are now (1994) about 370 home care teams of which over one-third are attached to hospice in-patient units.[15]

Thirdly, there are the symptom control teams which operate in hospitals and might consist of one or more special nursing sisters and a part-time consultant and social worker. They *advise* but on care given to patients in the wards. In January 1994 there were about 240 hospitals with such support teams or support nurses.[16]

Finally, there are now over 200 day hospices.

So from a few charitable hospices in the 1960s there are now a total of 203 in-patient units – including the continuing care units – providing more than 3,110 beds.[17] Of these, 153 are independent hospice units (including the Marie Curie and Sue Ryder Homes). There is an average of more than 49.1 beds per million population.[18]

The position now and the future

The growth of hospices, home care teams and support teams as outlined above was initiated by voluntary action and has been spasmodic, responding to perceived local need and demand. The national average disguises much variation, both regionally and between health districts, in the availability of services and the cover they offer. Regions such as Merseyside are well provided for, with 64.8 beds per million population, whereas others, such as Trent and Northern, have half this number, 32.6 and 32.2 beds per million respectively. Differences between individual district health authorities are just as great. Out of 180 English district health authorities, fifty-nine or just under one-third (32 per cent) do not have any hospice in-patient units of their own and rely on other districts for such services. The NE Thames Region, for example, which is where St Joseph's is, has 195 beds overall, that is 51.56 beds per million population, but six of its nine district health authorities do not have any in-patient beds of their own. This means that while beds may in theory be available, they are not necessarily near the people who need them. Their location is important both to the patients who are referred to them and the families and friends who want to visit. Some in-patient units are big, serving wide areas when what might be preferred are smaller local units easily reached by relatives and friends. Harold Allen turned down respite care in his local hospice, which would have given Lilian a much needed rest because he and Lilian felt it was just too far for her to travel every day (a six-mile bus journey on more than one bus). Arthur opted to go to his local hospital because it was just round the corner, familiar and convenient for his friendly neighbour and family to visit. It is clear that smaller units are needed serving local areas.

The range of home care provision is just as variable.[19] What constitutes a home care team in one area and how it operates can be quite different from what is found in another area. A survey conducted in 1990 showed that 46 per cent of teams had a doctor and 37 per cent had a social worker, but more than half of the 'teams' (55 per cent) consisted of just a single Macmillan nurse working alone.[20] A single unsupported nurse cannot provide the same kind of resources as a multi-disciplinary team. The needs of patients with terminal illness are numerous, requiring the skills of different professionals. A team is one way to achieve this.

Such is the St Joseph's Home Care Team, which is fully integrated with the work of the hospice and operates under the direction of its matron and medical director. It had a staff of three doctors, seven trained nurses, two social workers and a secretary, and serves the London Boroughs of Newham, Hackney and Tower Hamlets. A referred patient is visited and his or her needs assessed and then the frequency and nature of home visits are tailored to respond to the patient's needs, those of the family and the needs of the primary care team (GP and district nurses) which is looking after the patient. For patients and carers, the team is able to advise when needed, to supplement with hands-on care when primary care resources are overstretched, and step in when GPs show an unwillingness to visit.[21]

We saw in Chapter 5 how much value many patients put on seeing the same doctors and nurses. The trend amongst GPs to cut back on home visits[22] and the move amongst GPs to change their out-of-hours responsibilities[23] could make it more difficult for terminally ill patients at home who value seeing the same doctor and nurse. Terminally ill patients will need special provision if they are to remain at home rather than be admitted to hospital or hospice. The distinctive aspects of the St Joseph's Home Care Team which made such a difference for the patients and carers we visited were its multi-disciplinary character, the hands-on care which meant a nurse could step in and complement the services of the primary care team if needed and the twenty-four hour cover for which the team is unusual.[24] The significance of continuous cover for patients lay as much in the support it implied as in the practical help it offered. Presumably Dr Clayton was aware of this when he gave his home telephone number and bleeper number to Lilian Allen.[25] The continuity of staff, all of whom met the patient, and the twenty-four hour cover, gave security and peace of mind to patients and carers, enabling carers to cope at home when otherwise they might have agreed to a patient being admitted. Caring is a lonely, tiring and frightening job. Knowing there was someone at the end of a telephone to give advice meant carers felt able to carry on with their task. The number of people who can turn to relatives to help relieve the strain is few, especially if carers are elderly. This needs to be acknowledged in the nature of the support services for terminally ill people.

Hospices themselves touch only a small percentage of those who are dying,[26] St Joseph's catering for 15 per cent of the cancer deaths in its area. What happens to all those people with cancer who don't benefit from St Joseph's services and to most dying from other illnesses such as motor neurone disease or Alzheimer's disease? Authors of the Wilkes Report[27] hoped that the principles and practices of hospice care would be disseminated throughout services for terminally ill people without the need for further building of specialist in-patient units and the following decade saw a big expansion in the number of trained Macmillan nurses serving the community. In 1992 when there were 160,000 deaths from cancer, 100,000 patients were seen by hospices and palliative home care teams.[28] There has also been a slow but increasing ripple effect as the hospice ethic and skills have encouraged a review of all the services available to terminally ill people. Differences that were once very apparent between hospice and hospital are now not so marked. The challenge for the future is to show how the very high standards of hospice care can be brought to people in their own homes. Although people spend the larger part of their last year of life at home, they are not as visible there as when they are in institutions.[29] It is our view that the St Joseph's Home Care Team model, offering twenty-four hour cover and complementary support to the primary care team, is the best way of meeting the special needs of people who are dying at home and of their carers.

Hospice is no longer associated only with a building; it is a concept that can be brought to the care of the elderly, sick and dying in a number of settings. How this is done will depend on how services are conceived and developed and how the principles of cost-effectiveness are applied in the new purchaser and provider market. The reorganisation of the National Health Service means that hospices now compete alongside other agencies from the statutory and private sectors in getting money from district health authorities and local authorities. This market mechanism may undermine the holistic approach of hospice care because of the difficulties in demonstrating the cost-effectiveness of support and counselling services to the social and emotional well-being

of patients and families.[30] Cost-effectiveness and dying do not go
well together. We say this because in the reformed NHS more
and more emphasis is being put on primary care teams of GPs,
district nurses and social workers. They are supposed to offer the
main support to terminally ill people as well as other patients
who are at home and the hospice home care teams are to be
more and more limited to advice. While every effort should
be made to disseminate the specialist skills and knowledge of
hospice staff to a wider professional group, this should not be
done at the expense of a patient's access to those specialists. We
can only hope that it will be recognised that terminally ill people
need more than GPs and district nurses, who are generalists, can
offer. The terminally ill also need hands-on nursing from specialists in palliative medicine.

The future does not only lie with the Macmillan type of service
as the following examples illustrate. The Paddington Community
Hospital houses a Palliative Care Unit which is an NHS-funded
seventeen-bed unit for respite care, terminal care and symptom
control and is much used by local GPs, for cancer relief amongst
other purposes, and there are home care teams working from the
unit for cancer-related illnesses. There is also a 'hospice at home'
scheme for HIV/Aids patients which has three in-patient beds;
this scheme offers nursing care in addition to the usual palliative
care services in the community at whatever level the patient
needs up to twenty-four hours.

The caring-at-home principle is taken a step further by the
Peterborough Hospital-at-Home,[31] set up in 1978 and modelled
on a French hospital that had been running in Paris and Bayonne.
Patients with certain conditions who would otherwise be hospital-
ised can be admitted to the scheme and cared for at home.
Approximately half the patients are people returning home early
after surgery and the others are people with such conditions as
acute chest infections, cerebrovascular accidents and Aids which
require intensive nursing care. General practitioners take responsibility for patients and nursing care is given by the District
Nursing Service which in turn calls on Hospital-at-Home contrac-
ted staff to meet the patient's needs, visiting at least twice a day
over a twenty-four hour period. Volunteer patient aides are also
called on to help with practical and social needs. At the moment
Hospital-at-Home is the only scheme of its kind in Britain. The
majority of patients are elderly and many are terminally ill.

Half way between full home care and hospital care are small units such as the one in Doncaster to which patients are admitted to give carers short-term respite. 'Patients should be elderly people receiving care at home from community nurses whose carers need relief on a planned basis to alleviate stress or because of a temporary crisis.'[32] The Lambeth Community Care Centre[33] is run by a new breed of GPs. A new building, the centre was purpose-built to a domestic scale and opened in 1985 on the site of the old Lambeth General Hospital. The twenty beds are given to acute care, rehabilitation, respite care and palliative care. Patients from a small catchment area are referred by local GPs who have twenty-four hour responsibility for their patients on the wards. This means patients are never seen by deputising services but always by a known doctor. The wards are staffed by trained nurses. Not surprisingly, patients like it and GPs do as well because they can stay with their patient instead of passing them to a hospital or hospice. Each patient has a key worker from amongst the staff at the centre and is involved in their own 'care-plan'. Patients administer their own medication and are given their own notes and encouraged to read them. Cottage hospitals looking for a new role might consider Lambeth Community Care Centre while remembering that the commitment and dedication of its GPs is a condition of its success.

While it is to be hoped that some of the principles and practices that have evolved to care for those with cancer can be applied for the benefit of others with chronic and serious illness[34] this should not be at the cost of focused services for those in the final stages of a terminal illness and their carers.

Appendix III
Information about services

Some of this information is taken from the helpful appendix compiled by Colin Murray Parkes in his booklet 'Facing Death' published by the National Extension College.

1 For information about hospices and similar units, home care facilities and Macmillan services

i   *The Directory of Hospice Services in the UK and the Republic of Ireland*, published annually by St Christopher's Hospice Information Service, St Christopher's Hospice, 51–59 Lawrie Park Road, Sydenham, London SE26 6DU, Tel. 0181–778–9252. This is an invaluable reference book (available for the cost of the postage) in which people can see listed the hospice or hospice-type services available in their area. The directory lists all hospice and continuing care in-patient units including Sue Ryder Homes and Marie Curie Cancer Homes and children's hospices, home care teams and hospital support teams and all Macmillan services. The information officer at St Christopher's Hospice can help with enquiries.

Admission to a hospice or referral to a home care team, hospital support team or Macmillan service is normally arranged by a patient's GP or hospital doctor. While most hospices have a catchment area it may not be confined to one county. There is usually no charge for admission though a small number of units with no statutory funding may request a contribution towards patient care.

ii   *Cancer Relief Macmillan Fund, Anchor House, 15–19 Britten*

Street, London SW3 3TY, Tel. 0171–351–7811. Works to improve the quality of life for people with cancer and their families. It builds units for in-patients and day care and Macmillan nurses specially trained in cancer care give support and advice in the home-based services listed in the Directory of Hospices. Referral is usually via a GP, district nurse or hospital consultant.

iii *Marie Curie Cancer Care, Head Office, 28 Belgrave Square, London SW1X 8QG, Tel. 0171–235–3325. Scottish Office, 21 Rutland Street, Edinburgh EH1 2AH, Tel. 0131–229–8332.* Has eleven homes or hospice centres and nearly 5,000 part-time nurses who nurse patients in their own homes. The service is free of charge and gives a lot of assistance with night nursing. Referral is normally by a district nurse or sometimes a patient's GP or hospital consultant.

iv *Sue Ryder Foundation, Sue Ryder Home, Cavendish, Sudbury, Suffolk, CO10 8AY, Tel. 0178–728–0252.* Homes provide in-patient care for patients with a wide range of disabilities including some homes for patients with advanced cancer.

2 For medical help

i Phone your local *General Practitioner*. If you are not registered with a GP you can phone any GP (look in the Yellow Pages of the telephone directory under Doctors, Medical Practitioners), but you will not get help over the telephone.

ii If you are having problems, contact your local *Family Health Service Authority* (listed in the telephone directory) which produces a local health directory with a list of practitioners. This list is also available from your local *Community Health Council* and may be found in local libraries, post offices and pharmacies. In Scotland contact your local *Health Council* (look in the telephone directory).

iii In an emergency, phone 999 and ask for an ambulance.

3 **For information about some serious illnesses**

i *Aids*

ACET (Aids Care, Education and Training), PO Box 3693, London SW15 2BQ. National and international charity giving home care support and running educational programmes for young people.

National AIDS Helpline. Tel. 0800–567123 for free and confidential advice from trained advisers on all aspects of HIV and Aids and hospitals and hospices. Leaflets and booklets also available.

The Terrence Higgins Trust, 52–54 Gray's Inn Road, London WC1X 8JU. Helpline 0171–242–1010 offers welfare, legal and counselling help to people with Aids and HIV and their families. Practical help includes 'buddies' and support groups for people with Aids.

ii *Cancer*

BACUP, 3 Bath Place, Rivington Street, London EC2A 3JR, Tel. 0171–613–2121. A national cancer information service providing information, advice and support to cancer patients, their families and friends, health professionals and the general public by telephone or letter. Publications on most types of cancer produced in easy to understand language and available free of charge to individuals.

Cancerlink, 17 Britannia Street, London WC1X 9JN, Tel. 0171–833–2451. A national organisation offering a telephone and letter-answering service and range of publications on practical and emotional issues about cancer. People are invited to talk through what they want to know and staff are able to direct them to voluntary bodies and local organisations in their own area that may be able to help: special help available for ethnic minorities. Acts as a resource to a network of individuals and cancer self-help and support groups.

iii **Heart**

The Chest, Heart and Stroke Association, CHSA House, Whitecross Street, London SE1, Tel. 0171–490–7999, works to prevent strokes, helps those who have suffered strokes and their families and produces publications.

The British Heart Foundation, 14 Fitzhardinge Street, London W1H 4DH, Tel. 0171–935–0185, offers advice and information.

Other helpful organisations are listed in DSS Leaflet FB31, 'Caring for Someone'. A good reference book for voluntary organisations which should be available in public libraries is *The Voluntary Agencies Directory*, 1995/96, price £15.95, published and available from the National Council for Voluntary Organisations, Regent's Wharf, All Saints Street, London N1 9RL, Tel. 0171–713–6161.

4   For information about services, social support and financial help for the seriously ill and their carers

In April 1993, local authorities assumed full responsibility for supplying and funding care services as laid down in the Community Care Act 1990. Social service departments should have a home care department or its equivalent which coordinates provision once a client, GP or district nurse has contacted them. Social services work with area health authorities with the intention of providing a system of total care for the client. If you want to ask about receiving help in the home for a patient or their carer, your local social service department will be found in the telephone directory under the name of the council. Your GP should be familiar with all the services that are on offer and who to contact. Any service will probably depend on a 'needs assessment' being made by a visiting occupational therapist or social worker, possibly with advice from the GP or district nurse.

There are a number of *aids and adaptations* to the home that may be provided by social services such as wheelchairs, hoists, ripple mattresses, rubber sheets and sheepskins and, if necessary, physical adaptations to the home including rails, stair lifts and showers. What exactly they have will only be found out if a patient or carer enquire themselves of the social services or if their GP, district nurse or other person enquires for them.

Services include *home helps* (who may clean or shop for those living alone) and *meals on wheels* which will normally supply one hot meal a day from Monday to Friday.

Financial assistance can come from the government's Department of Social Security. A small booklet FB28 called 'Sick or Disabled' is a general guide to benefit entitlement for people who are sick or disabled for a few days or more. Further information can be found on DSS Freeline 0800–666–555, but they will not be able to advise on individual cases. You can get leaflets from your post office, otherwise your local social security office will have them (listed in the telephone book under Social Security or Benefits Agency) or you can write to Leaflets Unit, PO Box 21, Stanmore, Middlesex HA7 1AY.

Terminally ill patients who are 65 or over can now get an *attendance allowance* under the special rules introduced in October 1990, even if living alone. Terminal illness here is taken to mean that a person may not live longer than six months. The allowance does not depend on National Insurance contributions and is tax free. There are two rates depending on whether a patient needs to be looked after all day, all night or both. Patients need to get a report from their doctor and send it in with their claim which will be dealt with immediately. Information is in Leaflet DS 702 from local social security offices and post offices.

Social services also provide financial assistance in the form of travel permits (reduced fares on London Transport), a taxi-card scheme, safe-and-sound alarms and payments towards telephone rentals. Councils and areas within them operate differently and have slightly different services on offer, some of which are chargeable. Services are sometimes advertised by the council providing them but the onus may be on the client or carer to ask social services about them. The taxi-card system, for example, operates in all boroughs except Barnet, Greenwich, Redbridge and Westminster and is a scheme by which people who are unable to use public transport can make use of specified black cabs at a considerably reduced rate. The scheme is paid for mainly by the councils using it with nominal contributions from card holders. It is within an individual council's discretion as to how many people it accepts on the scheme and to whom it gives priority. Individual councils should be asked for information.

5   Information for carers

i   There is a helpful leaflet called 'Caring for Someone', FB31, available from local social security offices and main post offices. It outlines the benefits available to the carer and the person being cared for, the services on offer, where to go for them and useful phone numbers and addresses of organisations offering information and help to carers.

ii   *Carers National Association, 20–25 Glasshouse Yard, London EC1A 4JS, Tel. 0171–490–8818, and 11 Queen's Crescent, Glasgow G4 9AS, Tel. 0141–333–9495.* Campaigns for better benefits and services for carers. It is a voluntary organisation offering information and support to people who are caring at home as well as advice and information through a wide range of leaflets, one of which is 'Finding Your Way Around Benefits' (free). Branches throughout the country, details of which can be got from head office.

iii   *Association of CROSSROADS CARE Attendant Schemes, 10 Regent Place, Rugby, Warwickshire, CV21 2PN, Tel. 01788–573–653.* Provides care attendants in some districts who come into the home to give the carer a break. There are ten regional offices and 180 schemes throughout England, Scotland and Wales, details of which can be obtained from head office. Some schemes may have to make a nominal charge.

6   General information and advice

i   *Citizen's Advice Bureaux* or other local advice centres can advise on many problems, show you what is available in your area, who to contact and assist you if you are having difficulties or need help quickly. Your local branch will be listed in the telephone book or in Yellow Pages under 'Social Services and Welfare Organisations'.

ii   *Age Concern*, Astral House, 1268 London Road, London SW16 4EJ, Tel. 0181–679–8000. Offers support for older people and those who care for them with local groups providing services. Your local group will be listed in the telephone directory under Age Concern.

iii *Help the Aged*, 16–18 St James's Walk, London EC1R OBE, Tel. 0171–253–0253. Raises funds for projects and provides an advice service for the elderly and their carers.

iv   Your local church, synagogue, mosque or other religious organisation should be willing to offer consolation and advice. Even if you are not a practising member of any faith, you may find helpful priests and their equivalents.

7 When there is a death

i   You need to contact the Registrar of Births and Deaths. Deaths have to be registered in the local office covering the area in which the death occurred. A list of the addresses and telephone numbers of local registry offices is usually displayed in post offices, public libraries, other public buildings, doctors' surgeries and in the telephone directory.

ii   'What to do after a death', leaflet D49, is a Department of Social Security guide to what you must do and the help you can get and is available from any social security office or by post from Leaflets Unit, PO Box 21, Stanmore, Middlesex HA7 1AY.

iii 'Help when someone dies', leaflet FB29, advises on how to claim financial help towards the cost of a funeral, and on the help for widows, widowers and other relatives, one-parent families and guardians that is available.

8 To arrange a funeral

i   'What to do after a death', leaflet D49, advises what to do. Also helpful is the Which Consumers' Guide, 'What to do when someone dies', P. Harris, Which Books, revised edition, 1994.

ii   *Funeral directors* are listed in the Yellow Pages of the telephone directory. Of the trade associations, the oldest is the National Association of Funeral Directors, 618 Warwick Road, Solihull, West Midlands B91 1AA, Tel. 0121–711–1343, which has a code of practice which members must follow. There is also the British Institute of Funeral Directors, c/o Levertons, 212 Eversholt Street, London NW1 1BD, Tel.

0171–387–6075, and the Society of Allied and Independent Funeral Directors, c/o T. Cribb and Sons, 112 Rathbone Street, Canning Town, London E16 1JQ. In 1994 the Funerals Standards Council was formed, and can be contacted at 30 North Road, Cardiff CF1 3DY, Tel. 0122–238–2046, and a substantial number of funeral directors joined, mostly co-operatives.

iii *The British Humanist Association*, 14 Lamb's Conduit Passage, London WC1R 4RH, Tel. 0171–430–0908, can provide officiants for non-religious ceremonies.

iv *The Natural Death Centre*, 20 Heber Road, London NW2 6AA, Tel. 0181–208–2853, is an educational charity addressing how people might prepare for death and will advise on how to organise a funeral without using undertakers.

9 For advice and counselling

i *The National Association of Bereavement Services*, 122 Whitechapel, London E1 7PT, Tel. 0171–247–0617, is a support organisation for bereavement services and works with professionals to promote standards and training. It has produced a directory of services and has a helpline, Tel. 0171–247–1080, which can put bereaved and grieving people in touch with their most appropriate local service.

ii *CRUSE*, Bereavement Care, 126 Sheen Road, Richmond, TW9 1UR, Tel. 0181–940–4818, offers help on a national basis through local branches to bereaved individuals of all nationalities and beliefs. It offers counselling for the individual and for groups, advice and information on practical matters and opportunities for contact with others.

iii *The National Association of Widows*, 54–57 Allison Street, Digbeth, Birmingham B5 5TH, Tel. 0121–643–8348, offers advice and supportive friendship to widows.

iv *Society of Compassionate Friends*, 6 Denmark Street, Bristol BS1 5DQ, Tel. 0117–953–9639, offers friendship and understanding to bereaved parents.

What stands out from this listing is how much information is available to the assiduous seeker, and also how complex it all can be. If you are unsure where to go, the best general advice is from the local Citizen's Advice Bureau.

The special hardships of some people from ethnic minorities who do not speak English has been mentioned before. These have been reduced in the growing number of hospitals, health centres and GP surgeries which subscribe to Language Line, a new telephone interpreting service started from the Institute of Community Studies. Language Line provides immediate availability over the phone to interpreters in 140 different languages. Would-be users should apply to Jonathan O'Keefe at *Language Line*, 18 Victoria Park Square, London E2 9PF, Tel. 0181 983 4042.

Advice on living wills or 'advance directives' can be got from the Terrence Higgins Trust and the Voluntary Euthanasia Society.

Appendix IV
National Funerals College

The functions of a funeral are several. Speaking with the bereaved in our small study we were made aware of the funeral's importance as a public statement about the life of the deceased and as a final farewell for the survivors. But some services lamentably failed to do justice to the life of the deceased. Rather than feeling supported and comforted, some mourners were left disappointed and troubled by the funeral as well as by their loss. For close relatives the funeral marks the beginning of a new period in their lives. If it fails to mark both the uniqueness of the loss and its communality, the task of those grieving must be made that much more difficult. Numerous social changes, such as dying in institutions rather than at home, amalgamations and reorganisation in funeral directing, the popularity of cremation and the local authority's relationship to cemeteries and crematoria, have combined with changes in family and neighbourhood composition and the part played by religion to help shape funerals which for many are far from satisfactory.

Decisions about a funeral are usually taken when the bereaved are most distracted and distressed and least able to think through what they want and why. They are likely to refer choices to the funeral director (not now called a director for nothing) who in turn is likely to guide people to the most popular choices when perhaps what is needed is a question, namely what should be special about this occasion and why? If the question is put and answered, each funeral is likely to become a unique event marking a unique life. If funerals were more often thought of as the celebration of a life as well as a final parting, people might be willing to think about them more often in advance of death.

The evident need for improvement has led the authors to set

up the National Funerals College and invite a small group to guide it. The College is working to bring together several professional groups to see how they might do it better. One important condition for improvement is that funeral directors, crematorium managers, the clergy and bereavement counsellors should understand each other's roles better. Funerals have not always been conducted the way the majority are today. Their history is a testimony to the possibility of change in the future and it is change which the College is looking to bring about, keeping the needs of the deceased and his or her survivors to the forefront.

Short courses for local personnel are now being run around the country by the National Funerals College to bring together local clergy, funeral directors, crematorium managers and bereavement services and to start a dialogue about what improvements they might initiate locally. The possible changes in one area may not be so appropriate in another. It is hoped that these groups will become nuclei of reference for information and ideas on improvements to their local services and that their ideas can be shared with others through newsletters. The courses will help towards the production of material which will form the basis of an open distance learning scheme for all those servicing funerals. Before too long the public should be able to seek out the services of professionals who have been accredited with having attended or completed one of the National Funerals College's courses.

Some improvements will only follow on demand. So at the same time the College has drawn up a charter of 'rights' for the consumer, called The Dead Citizens Charter, so that any client arranging a funeral can easily familiarise him or herself with information on what should be possible and how they might go about achieving it. The charter will help focus people's attention before a funeral on the choices available, their rights and the maintenance of good standards. At the moment people are quite naturally reluctant to question the value and quality of service they have been given after the event; it is too upsetting to do so.

Further information can be obtained from The Reverend Dr Peter Jupp, Director, The National Funerals College, Braddan House, High Street, Duddington, Stamford, Lincs PE9 3QE. Professor Malcolm Johnson has taken over as chairman from Michael Young.

Notes

1 SLOW DEATH

1 *Social Trends*, Table 1.2, Age sex structure of the population, London, HMSO, 1990, p. 24.
2 E. Grundy, 'Future patterns of morbidity in old age', in F.I. Caird and J. Grimley Evans (eds), *Advanced Geriatric Medicine*, Bristol, John Wright, 1987.
3 *Review of National Cancer Registration System*, Series MB1, no. 17, London, OPCS, 1990.
4 Proponents of a 'compression of morbidity' have suggested that a near horizontal line of low mortality through all ages would be followed by a sharp drop at the age of 'natural death'. J.F. Fries, 'Aging, natural death, and the compression of morbidity', *New England Journal of Medicine*, 1980, vol. 303, no. 3, pp. 130–5. The facts have not borne out this argument. An alternative forecast of a 'pandemic of morbidity', especially of mental disorders, has been made by Dr Gruenberg. E. Gruenberg, 'The failures of success', *Health and Society*, Milbank Memorial Fund Quarterly, 1977, vol. 55, no. 1.
5 P. Ariès, *The Hour of Our Death*, Harmondsworth, Penguin, 1983.
6 N. Kfir and M. Slevin, *Challenging Cancer – From Chaos to Control*, London, Tavistock/Routledge, 1991, p. 53.
7 C.M. Parkes and R.S. Weiss, *Recovery from Bereavement*, New York, Basic Books, 1983, p. 17.
8 Anthony Clare, Foreword to Kfir and Slevin, *Challenging Cancer*.
9 P. Marris, *Widows and their Families*, London, Routledge & Kegan Paul, 1958. This was followed, in many British and US editions, by his *Loss and Change*, London, Routledge & Kegan Paul, revised edition, 1986.
10 M. Young, B. Benjamin and C. Wallis, 'Mortality of widowers', *Lancet*, 1963, vol. 2, pp. 454–6.
11 C.M. Parkes, B. Benjamin and R.G. Fitzgerald, 'Broken heart: a statistical study of increased mortality among widowers', *British Medical Journal*, 1969, vol. 1, pp. 740–3.
12 S. Frankel and D. Smith, 'Conjugal bereavement among the Huli

people of Papua, New Guinea', *British Journal of Psychiatry*, 1982, vol. 141, pp. 302–5.

13 M. Young, *The Metronomic Society*, London, Thames and Hudson, 1988 and M. Young and T. Schuller, *Life After Work*, London, HarperCollins, 1991.

14 For a history of St Joseph's Hospice and an outline of hospice work, see Appendix II.

15 Some of the differences between cancers and their associated survival probabilities are given in *Understanding Cancer*, London, Consumers' Association, Which Books, 1986. Profesor Nias in the foreword refers to the tremendous progress already made this century, 'from curing less than 5% of all cancers in 1900 to over 50% in 1985'.

16 The patients themselves frequently referred to the nurses in this team as Macmillan nurses (see Appendix II for information), so the term appears in some of the quotations. Home Care Team with capital letters is intended to distinguish the St Joseph's Home Care Team from more general home care services including home helps that may be provided by Social Service departments. The terminology has changed in the course of our enquiry. The National Health Service has taken over.

2 THE PATIENTS

1 A list of the informants and references to the pages where summary descriptions of them first appear in this chapter are given in Appendix I. This is for readers who at later stages want to refer back in order to see who people are.

2 The ages given in the summaries of people are the age when they died.

3 On the basis of her experiences and conversations with over 200 dying patients in a Chicago hospital. E. Kübler-Ross, *On Death and Dying*, London, Tavistock/Routledge, 1973.

4 C.M. Parkes, Foreword to Kübler-Ross, *On Death and Dying*.

5 T. Walter, *The Revival of Death*, London, Routledge, 1994.

6 E. Goffman, *Asylums*, New York, Anchor Books, 1961, p. 14.

7 'Women ... were less likely to die in their own homes, 20% compared with 30% for men, and more likely to die in a residential home, 21% against 4%.' A. Cartwright, 'The role of hospitals in caring for people in the last year of their lives', *Age and Ageing*, 1991, vol. 20, no. 4, pp. 271–4.

8 A.D. Weisman and J.W. Worden, 'Psychosocial analysis of cancer deaths', *Omega*, 1975, vol. 6, no. 1, pp. 61–75.

9 'Victor Marshall found that elderly respondents reported a desire to live in order to take care of another relative, usually a spouse, although the relationship occasionally was one between siblings or an adult child. Knowing that their relative could not live without them gave these people a reason to live.' K. Charmaz, *The Social Reality of Death*, Reading, MS, Addison–Wesley, 1980, p. 156 quoting

V. Marshall, 'Secularisation for impending death', *American Journal of Sociology*, 1975, vol. 80, pp. 1124–44.

10 M. Young and T. Schuller, *Life After Work*, London, HarperCollins, 1991.

11 W. Shakespeare, *King Lear*, v.ii.9.

12 C.M. Parkes makes similar observations in *Bereavement: Studies of Grief in Adult Life*, Harmondsworth, Penguin, 1972, pp. 102 and 106.

13 H. Beach, 'Sister death', in J. Neuberger and J.A. White (eds), *A Necessary End – Attitudes to Death*, London, Macmillan, Papermac, 1991, p. 25.

14 C.M. Parkes observes 'Panic attacks . . . were brought on by reminders of death and by lonelinesss at loss of support, and included "choking sensations", breathless attacks and other somatic expressions of fear.' *Bereavement: Studies of Grief in Adult Life*, p. 128.

15 John Donne, *Holy Sonnets*, vii.

3 THE BATTLE FOR INDEPENDENCE

1 C. Saunders, 'The treatment of intractable pain', *Proceedings of the Royal Society of Medicine*, March 1963, vol. 56, no. 3.

2 'Ideas about the future may have had only a tenuous link with reality and yet still be experienced as great loss if they can no longer be believed.' G.W. Brown and T. Harris, *Social Origins of Depression: A Study of Psychiatric Disorder in Women*, London, Tavistock, 1978, p. 234.

3 B. Inglis, *The Diseases of Civilisation*, London, Granada, A Paladin Book, 1983, p. 47.

4 C. Murray Parkes, 'Psycho-social transitions: a field for study', *Social Science and Medicine*, 1971, vol. 5, pp. 101–15.

5 Murray Parkes, 'Psycho-social transitions: a field for study', p. 102.

6 V. Clement-Jones, 'Cancer and beyond: the formation of BACUP', *British Medical Journal*, 1985, vol. 219, pp. 1021–23.

7 C.M. Parkes and R.S. Weiss, *Recovery from Bereavement*, New York, Basic Books, 1983.

8 See S. Greer and M. Watson, 'Mental adjustment to cancer: its measurement and prognostic importance', *Cancer Surveys*, 1987, vol. 6, no. 3.

9 E. Wilkes, 'Terminal care: how can we do better?', *Journal of the Royal College of Physicians of London*, 1986, vol. 20, no. 3, pp. 216–18.

10 P. Marris, *Loss and Change*, London, Routledge & Kegan Paul, revised edition, 1986, p. 6.

4 THE CARER AT HOME

1 D.W. Winnicott, *Collected Papers: Through Paediatrics to Psycho-analysis*, London, Tavistock Publications, 1958, p. 99.

2 A. Cartwright, 'The role of hospitals in caring for people in the last year of their lives', *Age and Ageing*, 1991, vol. 20, no. 4, pp. 271–4.

3 B. Jordan, *Value for Caring: Recognising Unpaid Carers*, Kings Fund Project Paper, 1990, no. 81, p. 16.

4 See J. Finch and J. Mason, *Negotiating Family Responsibilities*, London, Tavistock/Routledge, 1993.

5 S. Thompson and J. Kahn, *The Group Process and Family Therapy*, Oxford, Pergamon Press, 1988, p. 157.

6 J. Hinton, 'The influence of previous personality on reactions to having terminal cancer', *Omega*, 1975, vol. 6, no. 2, p. 109.

7 M. Young and P. Willmott, *Family and Kinship in East London*, Harmondsworth, Penguin, 1986; P. Townsend, *The Family Life of Old People*, London, Routledge & Kegan Paul, 1957.

8 A listing of services available to patients at home is in Appendix III.

9 J. Townsend, A.O. Frank, D. Fermont, S. Dyer, O. Karren, A. Walgrove and M. Piper, 'Terminal cancer care, and patients' preference for place of death: a prospective study', *British Medical Journal*, 1990, vol. 301. K.P. Dunphy and B.D.W. Amesbury in 'A comparison of hospice and home care patients: patterns of referral, patients' characteristics and predictors of place of death' came to the same sort of conclusion, *Palliative Medicine*, 1990, vol. 4, no. 2, pp. 105–11.

10 C. Murray Parkes, 'Terminal care: home, hospital or hospice?', *Lancet*, 1985, 19 January, pp. 155–7.

11 E. Wilkes, 'Dying now', *Lancet*, 1984, 28 April, pp. 950–2.

12 *Caring for People: Community Care in the Next Decade and Beyond*, London, HMSO, 1989, para. 8.35.

13 N. Mays, 'Community care', in G. Scambler (ed.), *Sociology as Applied to Medicine*, London, Bailliere Tindall, 1991, p. 242.

14 'Place of death', *Fact Sheet 7*, 1994, The Hospice Information Service, St Christopher's Hospice, derived from OPCS statistics.

15 Some of the main reasons given in another study for admitting the patient to hospital were that the relatives felt physically or emotionally unable to cope at home. Wilkes, 'Dying now'. Respite care can make a difference. Forty-two per cent of clients of St Christopher's Home Care Team died at home. Following the introduction of respite care in 1994–5, the figure increased to 49.5 per cent (personal communication).

16 'What little evidence that does exist would suggest major problems with the health of carers as they struggle themselves to cope with an illness that is located in another's body.' D. Armstrong, *An Outline of Sociology as Applied to Medicine*, London, Wright, 1989, p. 67, referring to J. Lewis and B. Meredith, 'Daughters caring for mothers: the experience of caring and its implications for professional helpers', *Ageing and Society*, 1988, vol. 8, pp. 1–21.

17 Dora's friend with whom she had planned to go on holiday (see Chapter 2).

18 But Hinton reminds us that 'calm is not the only appropriate emotion for dying'. 'Comparison of places and policies for terminal care', *The Lancet*, 1979, 6 January, pp. 29–32.

19 C. Seale and J. Addington-Hall, 'Dying at the best time', *Social Science and Medicine*, 1995, vol. 40, no. 5, pp. 589–95.

20 Tony Walter in a personal communication.

5   THE DOCTOR

1 S.B. Nuland, *How We Die*, London, Chatto & Windus, 1994, p. 43.
2 Quoted in Nuland, *How We Die*, p. 223.
3 Observations in some Scottish hospitals showed how much neglect of dying people there can be. 'Contact between nurses and the dying patients was minimal; distancing and isolation of patients by most medical and nursing staff were evident; this isolation increased as death approached.' M. Mills, H.T.O. Davies and W.A. Macrae, 'Care of dying patients in hospital', *British Medical Journal*, 1994, vol. 309, 3 September, pp. 583–6.
4 Quoted in *Death and Dying*, Workbook 2, Preparing for Death, Milton Keynes, Open University, 1992, p. 42.
5 In a previous publication it was stated that 'Every doctor could also be a teacher. The best already are.' M. Young, 'The expectations of patients', in D.J. Pereira Gray (ed.), *The Medical Annual 1985 – The Yearbook of General Practice*, London, Wright, 1985.
6 F. Clough, 'The validation of meaning in illness-treatment situations', in D. Hall and M. Stacey (eds), *Beyond Separation*, Routledge & Kegan Paul, London, 1979; L. Wallace, 'Informed consent in elective surgery: the "therapeutic" value?', *Social Science and Medicine*, 1986, vol. 22, no. 1, pp. 29–33. Quoted in *Death and Dying*, p. 47. I.L. Janis found amongst patients undergoing major surgery 'that those who were given realistic information, together with emotional support in advance of surgery, adjusted more easily to the trauma than those who had not been warned.' I.L. Janis, *Psychological Stress: Psychoanalytic and Behavioural Studies of Surgical Patients*, London, Chapman and Hall, 1958. C.M. Parkes and R.S. Weiss, *Recovery from Bereavement*, New York, Basic Books, 1983, p. 233. According to Parkes, this type of anticipation is 'worry work', *Bereavement: Studies of Grief in Adult Life*, Harmondsworth, Penguin, 1972, p. 93.
7 Personal communication. The study was conducted from the Cancer Research Campaign Communication and Counselling Research Centre and summaries of findings are given in a letter to *The Lancet*, 1994, vol. 344, no. 8936, 3 December.
8 H.J. Henderson, *New England Journal of Medicine*, 1935, 112, 819. Quoted by Lord Justice Edmund Davies, 'The patient's right to know the truth', *Proceedings of the Royal Society of Medicine*, 1973, vol. 66, pp. 533–6, June.
9 I.O. Glick, R.S. Weiss and C.M. Parkes, *The First Year of Bereavement*, New York, John Wiley, 1974, p. 290.
10 P.Ariès, *The Hour of Our Death*, trans. H. Weaver, Harmondsworth, Penguin, 1983, p. 561. Tolstoy gives an example. 'What tormented Ivan Ilyich most was the pretence, the lie, which for some reason they all kept up, that he was merely ill and not dying.... And the pretence made him wretched.' Leo Tolstoy, *The Death of Ivan Ilyich*, Harmondsworth, Penguin Classics, 1989, p. 142. Cannadine has dis-

puted the dating. He says that 'the impact of the First World War on attitudes to death has been underrated by sociologists and historians'. 'War and death, grief and mourning in modern Britain' in J. Whaley (ed.), *Mirrors of Mortality: Studies in the Social History of Death*, London, Europa, 1981, p. 189.

11 G. Gorer, *Death, Grief and Mourning in Contemporary Britain*, London, Cresset Press, 1965, p. 171.
12 The practice seems to have been the same in Japan in the more recent past.

> The major feature in the Japanese treatment of cancer is that doctors do not tell the patient the 'verdict'. . . . When asked whether they would like to be told if they were victims, they responded almost unanimously that they would prefer not to be told. . . . One reason is almost always given for the current practice. Many people cite the immediate deterioration of patients who are accidentally told of the diagnosis, and claim that most humans are not strong enough to live with the notion of impending death.

The author explains that one of the reasons for concealment is related to the lifetime employment system in Japan; someone with cancer, if revealed, might be taken out of the normal career development path. E. Ohnuki-Tierney, *Illness and Culture in Contemporary Japan*, Cambridge, Cambridge University Press, 1984, pp. 62–6.
13 Cas Wouters, 'Changing regimes of power and emotions at the end of life: The Netherlands 1930–1990', *Netherlands Journal of Sociology*, 1990, vol. 26, Part II, pp. 151–67.
14 A. Cartwright, L. Hockey, J.L. Anderson, *Life Before Death*, Institute for Social Studies in Medical Care, London, Routledge & Kegan Paul, 1973, Chapter 9.
15 C. Seale, 'Communication and awareness about death', *Social Science and Medicine*, 1991, vol. 32, no. 8, pp. 943 and 948.
16 R. Williams, 'Social movements and disordered bodies: the reform of birth, sex, drink, and death in Britain since 1850', in C. Crouch and A. Heath (eds), *Social Research and Social Reform*, Oxford, Clarendon Press, 1992, p. 118.
17 Quoted in D.H. Novack, R. Plumer, R.L. Smith, H. Ochitill, G.R. Morrow and J.M. Bennett, 'Changes in physicians' attitudes toward telling the cancer patient', *Journal of the American Medical Association*, 1979, vol. 241, no. 9.
18 Novack *et al.*, 'Changes in physicians' attitudes'.
19 B. Glaser and A. Strauss, *Awareness of Dying*, London, Weidenfeld & Nicolson, 1966, p. 11.
20 J. Hinton, *Dying*, Harmondsworth, Penguin Books, 1990, p. 127.
21 C. Saunders, 'Telling patients', *District Nursing*, 1965, September.
22 E. Wilkes, 'Terminal care: how we can do better?', *Journal of Royal College of Physicians of London*, 1986, vol. 20, no. 3, pp. 216–18.
23 J. Townsend, A.O. Frank, D. Fermont, S. Dyer, O. Karren, A. Walgrove and M. Piper, 'Terminal cancer care and patients' preference

for place of death: a prospective study', *British Medical Journal*, 1990, vol. 301, pp. 415–17.

24 C.M. Parkes, 'Terminal care: home, hospital or hospice?', *Lancet*, 1985, 19 January, pp. 155–7.

25 Hospitals have been affected too. As far back as 1984 Parkes noted that improvement in pain control in a hospital might be attributed to the diffusion effect of the hospice skills. C.M. Parkes and J. Parkes, ' "Hospice" versus "hospital" care: re-evaluation after 10 years as seen by surviving spouse', *Postgraduate Medical Journal*, 1984, vol. 60, pp. 120–4.

26 C.M. Parkes, 'Psychological aspects' in C. Saunders (ed.), *The Management of Terminal Disease*, London, Edward Arnold, 1978, p. 53.

27 E. Kübler-Ross, *On Death and Dying*, London, Tavistock/Routledge, 1989, p. 246.

28 K. Sikora and H. Smedley, *Cancer*, London, Heinemann Medical Student Reviews, 1988, p. 11.

29 B. Davey, 'Ethical framework of the consultation: doctors' assumptions about the patient's need to know', paper given to the International Conference on Communication in Health Care, Churchill College, Cambridge, July 1988. See also R.S. Downie and K.C. Calman, *Healthy Respect: Ethics in Health Care*, London, Faber & Faber, 1987.

30 'People are not even to be told that they are dying, at the most extreme end of the spectrum, lest they stop fighting and therefore shorten their lives by a few hours or days.' J. Neuberger and J.A. White, *A Necessary End – Attitudes to Dying*, London, Macmillan, Papermac, 1994, p. 13.

31 L. Rentoul, 'The stress of communicating with bereaved relatives: an exploration of the view of doctors and nurses in medicine and surgery', paper presented to Leicester Conference on Death and Dying, 1993.

32 B. Davey, 'The nurses' dilemma: truthtelling or big white lies', in D. Dickenson and M. Johnson (eds), *Death, Dying and Bereavement*, London, Sage, 1993, pp. 116–23.

33 C. Seale, 'Communication and awareness about death: a study of a random sample of dying people', *Social Science and Medicine*, 1991, vol. 32, no. 8, pp. 943–52, p. 945.

34 R. Buckman, 'Breaking bad news: why is it still so difficult?', *British Medical Journal*, 1984, vol. 288, 26 May, pp. 1597–9.

35 N. Kfir and M. Slevin, *Challenging Cancer – From Chaos to Control*, London, Tavistock/Routledge, 1991, p. 7.

36 J. Hinton, *Dying*, Harmondsworth, Penguin Books, 1990, p. 135.

37 C.M. Parkes, 'Psychological aspects', in C.M. Saunders, (ed.), *The Management of Terminal Disease*, London, Edward Arnold, 1978, p. 48.

38 Hinton, *Dying*, p. 139.

39 It is perhaps fortunate that according to Parkes the predictions made by doctors are generally too favourable. They err towards optimism. See C.M. Parkes in symposium on 'The patient's right to know the

truth', *Proceedings of the Royal Society of Medicine*, 1973, vol. 66, June.

40 R. Lamerton, *East End Doc*, Cambridge, Lutterworth, 1986, p. 11.
41 'The adverse effects of poor communication are greatly exacerbated for those patients who do not speak English.' *What Seems to be the Matter: Communication Between Hospitals and Patients*, Audit Commission, London, HMSO, 1993, p. 53.
42 The issue is dealt with at length by R. Frankenberg (ed.), *Time, Health and Medicine*, London, Sage Publications, 1992.
43 Patients are often reluctant to raise new problems in case they turn out to be serious and involve yet more dreaded treatment. Usually called 'under-reporting', Cartwright noted this and said that 'when the doctor gave the impression that he was busy or uninterested it seemed that people were rather less likely to seek his advice'. A. Cartwright, L. Hockey and J.L. Anderson, *Life Before Death*, Institute for Social Studies in Medical Care, London, Routledge & Kegan Paul, 1973, p. 89.
44 D. Silverman, 'Going private: ceremonial forms in a private oncology clinic', *Sociology*, 1984, vol. 18, no. 2, pp. 191–204.
45 Charles Fletcher and Paul Freeling have gone far to work out such a policy in *Talking and Listening to Patients – A Modern Approach*, Nuffield Provincial Hospitals Trust, London, 1988.
46 Rentoul, 'The stress of communicating with bereaved relatives'.
47 S.J. Read, B.E. Hutchinson and N.M. Dennis, *Pre-discharge Communication Project*, Grantham and Kesteven General Hospital, College of Health, 1992.
48 This is also the conclusion of another study, B. Hogbin and L. Fallowfield, 'Getting it taped', *British Journal of Hospital Medicine*, 1989, vol. 41.
49 Quoted in Open University Workbook 2, *Death and Dying*, p. 42.
50 If children were taught more about their bodies – what is more obvious for an education than that? – it could remove some of the 'magic-bullet' power from doctors. Doctors have a remarkable lack of interest in health education which could reduce the number of their patients.

6 PAIN AND EUTHANASIA

1 C.M. Parkes, 'Psychological aspects', in C. Saunders (ed.), *The Management of Terminal Disease*, London, Edward Arnold, 1978, p. 49.
2 See L.D.L. Patrick and G. Scambler, *Sociology as Applied to Medicine*, London, Baillière's Concise Medical Textbooks, 1986, p. 104.
3 Degenaar argues for an interdisciplinary approach to pain which reflects its many-sidedness by unifying the way we consider pain in the body (the physical and physiological), and the person (the philosophical or meaning-given and social dimension of pain). J.J. Degenaar, 'Some philosophical considerations on pain', *Pain*, 1979, vol. 7, pp. 281–304.
4 It comes from the Latin word 'pallium', a cover or cloak. 'In the

hospice setting "palliative" refers to the control of symptoms by use of medications and non-pharmacological interventions.' R.J. Dunlop and J.M. Hockley (eds), *Terminal Care Support Teams: The Hospital –Hospice Interface*, Oxford, Oxford University Press, 1990, p. 83.

5 C. Saunders, 'Voluntary euthanasia', *Palliative Medicine*, 1992, vol. 6, no. 1, pp. 1–5.

6 R. G. Twycross, 'Euthanasia – a physician's viewpoint', based on a lecture given to the International Conference on Voluntary Euthanasia and Suicide, Oxford, 1980.

7 C. Seale and J. Addington-Hall, 'Euthanasia: why people want to die earlier', *Social Science and Medicine*, 1994, vol. 39, no. 5, pp. 647–54.

8 'Euthanasia: what is the good death?', *Economist*, 1991, 20 July, p. 21.

9 Institute of Medical Ethics Working Party on the Ethics of Prolonging Life and Assisting Death, *Lancet*, 1990, vol. 336, 8 September, p. 610.

10 Working Party to review the BMA guidance on euthanasia, *The Euthanasia Report*, BMA, The Chameleon Press, London, 1988.

11 Select Committee on Medical Ethics, House of Lords Session 1993–94, Vol. 1-Report, 1994.

12 Parliamentary Debates, House of Lords, Debate on Select Committee on Medical Ethics, vol. 554, no. 83, col. 1374, 9 May 1994.

13 World Health Organisation in 1992 (reinforcing what we already know for Britain) showed that people are reporting more frequent and longer lasting episodes of serious and acute illness than they did 60 years ago. 'The future of medicine', *Economist*, 1994, 19 March.

14 Many doctors also know of patients who seemed to have no chance of living, and yet lived. 'I have vivid and sobering memories of a man with lymphoma who went into a permanent remission after weeks of extremely unpleasant treatment which I had felt was totally unjustified. I was wrong and my boss was right and I get a Christmas card from the patient each year to remind me.' Dr Sheila Cassidy, 'The dignity of death', *Royal Society of Arts Journal*, 1994, vol. CXLII, no. 5451, July.

15 Seale and Addington-Hall, 'Euthanasia: why people want to die earlier'.

16 E. Durkheim, *Suicide*, London, Routledge & Kegan Paul, 1952, p. 209.

17 M. Young, B. Benjamin and C. Wallis, 'Mortality of widowers', *Lancet*, 1963, vol. 2, pp. 454–6.

18 B. Bettelheim, *The Informed Heart*, Harmondsworth, Penguin, 1986, p. xvi.

19 C. Seale and J. Addington-Hall, 'Dying at the best time', *Social Science and Medicine*, 1995, vol. 40, no. 5.

20 L. Kennedy, *Euthanasia: The Good Death*, London, Chatto & Windus, 1990, pp. 6–7.

21 I. Kennedy, 'The quality of mercy: patients, doctors and dying', The Upjohn Lecture at the Royal Society, 25 April, 1994. It has been pointed out to us that the words put into the mouth of Dr A. are misleading. Pain control is achieved by giving drugs and increasing the dosage until pain control is achieved and then the dose is kept

at this level, which can be well short of the level that would bring on death.
22 Kennedy, 'The quality of mercy'.
23 BMA Statement on Advance Directives, November 1992.
24 B.J. Ward and P.A. Tate, 'Attitudes among NHS doctors to requests for euthanasia', *British Medical Journal*, 1994, vol. 308, pp. 1332–4. They said of the 32 per cent proportion that it was 'comparable to the 29% of doctors in an Australian study who said that they had taken active steps to end a patient's life but smaller than the 41% of Dutch doctors who admitted having taken active steps in studies conducted in the Netherlands before the change in legislation in 1993'.

7 BEYOND OUR CARE BUT NOT OUR CARING

1 C.M. Parkes, 'Bereavement as a psychosocial transition: processes of adaptation to change', *Journal of Social Issues*, 1988, vol. 44, no. 3, pp. 53–65.
2 B. Raphael, *The Anatomy of Bereavement*, New York, Basic Books, 1983. Cited in C.M. Parkes, 'Research: bereavement', *Omega*, 1987–8, vol. 18, no. 4.
3 C.M. Parkes, *Bereavement: Studies of Grief in Adult Life*, Harmondsworth, Penguin, 1972, p. 93. 'Worry work' is a term coined by I.L. Janis in *Psychological Stress: Psychoanalytic and Behavioural Studies of Surgical Patients*, London, Chapman and Hall, 1958. Freud had a similar term, 'grief work', which he used in 'Mourning and melancholia', standard edition, vol. 14, 1971.
4 C.M. Parkes, 'Evaluation of a bereavement service', *Journal of Preventive Psychiatry*, 1981, vol. 1, no. 2.
5 Parkes, 'Bereavement as a psychosocial transition', p. 56.
6 J. Bowlby, *Attachment and Loss*, vol. 1, *Attachment*, London, Hogarth Press, 1969.
7 We are grateful to Sheila Thompson for discussing this point with us.
8 See J.W. Worden, *Grief Counselling and Grief Therapy*, London, Tavistock, 1983 and C.M. Parkes, *Bereavement: Studies of Grief*.
9 A.D. Weisman and J.W. Worden, 'Psychosocial analysis of cancer deaths', *Omega*, 1975, vol. 6, no. 1, pp. 61–75. F. Mansell Pattison, 'Psychosocial predictions of death prognosis', *Omega*, 1974, vol. 5, no. 2, 1974. A.A. Harrison and N.E.A. Kroll, 'Variations in death rates in the proximity of Christmas', *Omega*, 1985–6, vol. 16, no. 3.
10 C.M. Parkes and R.S. Weiss, *Recovery from Bereavement*, New York, 1983, p. 19.

8 THE AFTERLIFE

1 P. Rosenblatt, P. Walsh and D. Jackson, *Grief and Mourning in Cross-Cultural Perspective*, USA, H.R.A.F. Press, 1976, Chapter 3, p. 51.
2 J. Goody, *Death, Property and the Ancestors*, London, Tavistock, 1962, p. 371.

3 B. Malinowski, *Argonauts of the Western Pacific*, London, Routledge, 1922, p. 72.

4 R. Firth, *Rank and Religion in Tikopia*, London, Allen & Unwin, 1970, p. 75.

5 I.O. Glick, R.S. Weiss and C.M. Parkes, *The First Year of Bereavement*, New York, Wiley & Sons, 1974, suggest bereaved people in a study by Rees, 1971, might be reluctant to reveal information because they think it could be taken to indicate mental illness.

6 Parkes has said that the loss of an elderly parent is perhaps the least distressing bereavement. C.M. Parkes, *Bereavement: Studies of Grief in Adult Life*, Harmondsworth, Penguin, 1986, p. 141. But this is not necessarily true of any particular individual. A common reason for people to seek help from Cruse (a bereavement organisation) and from psychiatrists is the death of a parent in adult life.

7 G. Gorer, *Death, Grief, and Mourning in Contemporary Britain*, London, Cresset Press, 1965, Ch. 2.

8 Parkes, *Bereavement: Studies of Grief in Adult Life*, p. 68.

9 'In the case of domestic animals, separation from the human beings who care for them induces similar behaviour.' C.M. Parkes and R.S. Weiss, *Recovery from Bereavement*, New York, Basic Books, 1983, p. 3.

10 C.M. Parkes, 'Bereavement as a psychosocial transition: processes of adaptation to change', *Journal of Social Issues*, 1988, vol. 44, no. 3, pp. 53–65.

11 Glick, Weiss and Parkes, *The First Year of Bereavement*, p. 11.

12 Glick, Weiss and Parkes, p. 137.

13 In another study 'Almost half the people interviewed had hallucinations or illusions of the dead spouse.' W. Dewi Rees, 'The hallucinations of widowhood', *British Medical Journal*, 1971, vol. 4, pp. 39–41.

9 IN CONCLUSION: COLLECTIVE IMMORTALITY

1 M. Young, B. Benjamin and C. Wallis, 'Mortality of widowers', *Lancet*, 1963, vol. 2, pp. 454–6.

2 For a general review see C.M. Parkes, 'Research: bereavement', *Omega*, 1987–88, vol. 18, no. 4.

3 Parkes, 'Research: bereavement', p. 366.

4 Adam Smith, *The Theory of Moral Sentiments*, Oxford, Clarendon Press, 1976, p. 130.

5 E. Grundy, 'Future patterns of morbidity in old age', in F.I. Caird and J. Grimley Evans (eds), *Advanced Geriatric Medicine*, Bristol, Wright, 1987, p. 70.

6 Much will always depend on the personality of the doctor. In 1940 Churchill began a radio talk to the British people with the blunt words 'The news from France is very bad.' 'Confidence in him (and in ourselves) grew before he had said another word.' T.B. Brewin,

'The cancer patient: communication and morale', *British Medical Journal*, 1977, vol. 2, pp. 1623–7.

7 For a more general discussion see Appendix II.

8 Quoted in T. Walter, *The Revival of Death*, London, Routledge, 1994, p. 72.

9 The knowledge may not apply to the contacts which have to be made with the bureaucracy. The community with real people in it may not show much concern. But the giant bureaucracy of the unknown has to be kept fully informed. The government's booklet about death goes into immense detail. The Registrar of Births and Deaths will give you 'A Certificate for Burial or Cremation (known as the Green Form) unless the coroner has given you an Order for Burial (Form 101) or a Certificate for Cremation (Form E). These give permission for the body to be buried or for an application for cremation to be made. It should be taken to the funeral director so that the funeral can be held.' *What To Do After A Death*, London, HMSO, 1993, p.14. Father Time has many disguises!

10 T. Walter, *Funerals and How to Improve Them*, London, Hodder & Stoughton, 1990. J. Wynne Willson, *Funerals without God: A Practical Guide to Non-religious Funerals*, British Humanist Association, 1989, was written in very much the same vein.

11 T. Walter, *Funerals*, p. 218.

12 Described in Appendix IV.

13 Social and Community Planning Research, Dartmouth, November, 1992.

14 G. Gorer, *Death, Grief and Mourning in Contemporary Britain*, London, Cresset Press, 1965, p. 166.

15 D.J. Enright (ed.), *The Oxford Book of Death*, Oxford, Oxford University Press, 1983.

16 'The fact that a man as spirit often receives more deference from, and exerts greater power over, people than while living may explain the apparent absence of the fear of death that has been observed in some primitive and ancestor-worship societies.' Robert Blauner, 'Death and social structure', *Psychiatry*, 1966, vol. 29, pp. 378–94.

17 Lord Tennyson, 'Tithonus', 27.

18 L. Mumford, *The City in History*, Harmondsworth, Penguin, 1966, p. 14. He also remarks that Israel is claimed as a Jewish patrimony because that is where the sacred graves of the forefathers were situated.

19 R. Hertz, *Death and the Right Hand*, London, Cohen & West, 1960, p. 81.

20 Rabbi Albert Friedlander, in R. Dinnage (ed.) *The Ruffian on the Stair*, Harmondsworth, Penguin, 1992.

21 G. Manley Hopkins, 'Spring', *Selected Poems*, London, Heinemann, 1953.

22 This was urged by Gorer as a means of relieving some of the pain for the mourners who were also the carers. Gorer, *Death, Grief and Mourning*, p. 116.

23 R. Dawkins, *The Selfish Gene*, Oxford, Oxford University Press, 1989, pp. 34–5.
24 M. Holroyd, 'How do we block the drain?', *Times Literary Supplement*, 1995, 23 June.
25 We have been influenced by a treatment by two anthropologists, M. Bloch and J. Parry, *Death and the Regeneration of Life*, Cambridge, Cambridge University Press, 1982.
26 D. Hume, *Enquiries Concerning the Human Understanding and Concerning the Principles of Morals*, 2nd edn., Oxford, Clarendon Press, 1902, Section IX, Part 1, para. 222.
27 Bettelheim said that 'If there is a central theme to the wide variety of fairy tales, it is that of a rebirth to a higher plane.' B. Bettelheim, *From the Uses of Enchantment*, London, Thames & Hudson, 1976, p. 179.
28 Open University Course Workbook on *Death and Dying*, No. 1, p. 27.
29 'If conditions are wrong, the death of one can lead to the death of ten, the death of ten to the death of a hundred, and the death of a hundred to the kind of escalation whose effects already mar the history of mankind. But reactions may be of another sort entirely, including insistence that help be extended to the suffering, that killing end, that there be a stop to the making of victims. Out of the distress created in us by death and by grief may spring a discontent whose consequences are creative rather than destructive.' C.M. Parkes and R.S. Weiss, *Recovery from Bereavement*, New York, Basic Books,, 1983, p. 5.
30 Thomas Traherne, *The Preparative II*.
31 S. Freud, *Civilization and its Discontents*, London, Hogarth Press, 1929, p. 8.
32 I. Wilson, *The After Death Experience*, London, Corgi, 1990.
33 W. James, *The Varieties of Religious Experience*, New York, Longmans, 1902.
34 Lucretius quoted in Jane Wynne Willson, *Funerals Without God*, British Humanist Association, London, 1989, p. 47.

APPENDIX II

1 St Joseph's Hospice 82nd *Annual Report*.
2 C. Saunders, 'The evolution of the hospices' in R.D. Mann (ed.), *The History of the Management of Pain*, Parthenon Publishing Group, Carnforth, UK, 1988.
3 *Annual Report*, St Joseph's Hospice, 1991, p. 9.
4 *1994 Directory of Hospice and Palliative Care Services*, Hospice Information Service, St Christopher's Hospice, p. iv.
5 Definition by the National Council for Hospice and Specialist Palliative Care Services, *1994 Directory of Hospice and Palliative Care Services*.
6 *Cancer Relief – from Vision to Reality*, Information Sheet to mark 75th Anniversary, 1986.
7 Standing Medical Advisory Committee: Standing Sub-Committee on

Cancer: Wilkes Report on Terminal Care Services for Cancer, *Terminal Care – Report of a Working Group*, DHSS 1980.

8 This included the cost of specialist training.

9 *1993 Directory of Hospice Services*, Hospice Information Service, St Christopher's.

10 The people we talked to in East London often called the Home Care nurses from St Joseph's Hospice 'Macmillan nurses' although they are no longer funded by CRMF.

11 R.J. Dunlop and J.M. Hockley, *Terminal Care Support Teams: The Hospital–Hospice Interface*, Oxford Medical Publications, New York, Oxford University Press, 1990, p. 83.

12 Reviewing literature on the subject Clive Seale suggests that there are probably as many different types of hospice care as there are hospices. C.F. Seale, 'What happens in hospices: a review of research evidence', *Social Science and Medicine*, 1989, vol. 28, no. 6, pp. 551–9.

13 Marie Curie Cancer Care has eleven hospice centres in the UK and nine of these have Home Care teams attached. They also provide a nursing service in partnership with most health authorities from a bank of 5,000 part-time Marie Curie nurses who nurse patients in their own homes.

14 The Sue Ryder Foundation provides beds for patients with a wide range of disabilities including some homes specially for patients with cancer.

15 *1994 Directory of Hospice and Palliative Care Services*.

16 Ibid.

17 Ibid.

18 B. Lunt and R. Hillier, 'Terminal Care: present services and future priorities, *British Medical Journal*, 1981, vol. 283, pp. 595–8.

19 In 1985, Lunt observed that the imbalance between the south east and the rest of the country in Home Care support had been reduced, but that there were still large differences between regions though with no clear geographical trend. B. Lunt, 'Terminal cancer care services: recent changes in regional inequalities in Great Britain', *Social Science and Medicine*, 1985, vol. 20, no. 7, pp. 753–9.

20 A.M. Smith, A. Eve, N.P. Sykes, 'Palliative care service in Britain and Ireland 1990 – an overview', *Palliative Medicine*, 1992, vol. 6, pp. 277–91.

21 Some GPs of the patients we visited remained fully involved with the patient's care, such as Harold's Dr Clayton and Kenneth's Dr Norgrove. Others were less involved and some never visited their patients during the time we knew them, handing over responsibility totally to the St Joseph's Home Care Team.

22 'The decline in home visiting by general practitioners over the last quarter of a century (Cartwright and Anderson 1981) has come at a time when it is probably more needed by the housebound and seriously ill, as hospital stays have shortened and there is more and more emphasis on community care.' Ann Cartwright, *The Role of the General Practitioner in Caring for People in the Last Year of*

Their Lives, London, King Edward's Hospital Fund for London, 1990, p. 28.

23 'In a nationwide survey of G.P.s undertaken by the BMA's general medical services committee in 1992, 73% of G.P.s said they would like to opt out of the current 24-hour commitment.' A number of measures have been agreed between the BMA and the Department of Health. Deputies will be liable for their own acts and omissions and GPs will only be obliged to visit a patient at home during the night if travel by car or taxi could endanger the patient's health. There will still be home visits by GPs at night but GPs will be able to provide alternative out of hours care, such as all-night primary care emergency centres. *British Medical Association*, Press Release, 19 May 1994.

24 The Ellenor Foundation Home Care Service also provides a twenty-four hour on-call service for patients and their carers.

25 They were hardly used. Once or twice in the whole year that Harold was nursed at home a call was made and one of these calls was for assistance after Harold had died.

26 Statistics from the OPCS suggest that hospices together look after 12 per cent of all deaths and 18 per cent of cancer deaths. Table 14 Series DH1 and Table 7 Series DH1 no. 21, quoted in *Place of Death*, Fact Sheet 7, The Hospice Information Service.

27 Standing Medical Advisory Committee, *Terminal Care*.

28 The Hospice Information Service.

29 D. Clark, *Partners in Care: Hospices and Health Authorities*, Aldershot, Avebury, 1993.

30 'Among the elderly individuals living alone in the 900 strong sample used (mean age eighty-two), those who had had just standard hospital care were twice as likely to have gone back into hospital as those who had had post-discharge community support.' David Taylor, quoting from the Medical Research Council's Epidemiology and Medical Care Unit, *Hospital at Home: The Coming Revolution*, London, Kings Fund Centre Health and Social Care Communication, 1989, p.9.

31 C. Bunce, 'Hospital at home', *Fundholding*, 1993, vol. 2, no. 18 and Taylor, *Hospital at Home*.

32 J. Hughes and P. Gordon, *An Optimal Balance? – Primary Healthcare and Acute Hospital Services in London*, King's Fund London Initiative, Working Paper No. 8, London, King's Fund Centre, 1992. p. 30.

33 Gillian Wilce, *A Place Like Home: A Radical Experiment in Health Care*, London, Bedford Square Press, 1989. Lambeth Community Care Centre Philosophy Document and Fact Sheet. R. Higgs, 'Example of intermediate care: the new Lambeth Community Care Centre', *British Medical Journal*, 1985, vol. 291, pp. 1395–7.

34 'the needs of chronically ill, older patients who are less likely to have near relatives to care for them seem less likely to be met by either hospice or hospital services. These are the people who are most likely to be in residential nursing homes ... a careful evaluation of their possible needs should be made. ... It could be that they are being denied helpful therapy and skilled and specialized care from which

they would benefit.' Ann Cartwright, 'The role of hospitals in caring for people in the last year of their lives', *Age and Ageing*, 1991, vol. 20, no. 4, pp. 271–4.

Index